Management of Continence and
Urinary Catheter Care

Other books in the *BJN* monograph series:

Towards 2000: Perspectives on preregistration nurse education edited by Jeremy Pope Cruickshank, Martyn Bradbury and Steve Himsworth

Management in Nursing edited by Jane Fox and Dawn Forman

Aspects of Cardiovascular Nursing edited by Jeremy Pope Cruickshank, Martyn Bradbury and Steve Ashurst

Management of Continence and Urinary Catheter Care

BJN monograph

edited by
Jeremy Pope Cruickshank and Sue Woodward

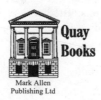

Quay
Books

Mark Allen
Publishing Ltd

Quay Books Division, Mark Allen Publishing Limited
Jesses Farm, Snow Hill, Dinton, Wiltshire, SP3 5HN

British Library Cataloguing-in-Publication Data
A catalogue record is available for this book

© Mark Allen Publishing Ltd 2001
ISBN 1 85642 201 1

Printed in the UK by Bath Press, Bath

Contents

Section four
Perspectives of education, research and audit

List of contributors

Freya Adams is Practice Development Nurse, Cardiology NDU, Addenbrooke's NHS Trust Hospital, Cambridge.

Ray Addison is Nurse Consultant in Bladder and Bowel Dysfunction, The Lancaster Suite, Mayday University Hospital, Croydon, Surrey.

Valerie Bayliss is Clinical Services Leader (Continence) North Hampshire PCT, Parklands Hospital, Basingstoke.

Ellen Carter is Senior Lecturer in Health and Community Studies, De Montfort University, Leicester, in conjunction with the Leicestershire MRC Incontinence Study Team.

Mary Cooke was formerly Head of Nursing and Midwifery Research, Homerton College, Central Nursing Department, Addenbrooke's NHS Trust Hospital, Cambridge.

Willie Doherty is Clinical Nurse Specialist, Park Drive Health Centre, Baldock, Herts.

Grace Dorey is Extended Scope Practitioner (Continence), North Devon District Hospital NHST, Barnstaple and Specialist Continence Physiotherapist Somerset Nuffield Hospital, Taunton.

Ann Evans is Research Nurse, Department of Urology, Southmead Hospital, North Bristol Healthcare Trust.

Dr Helen Godfrey is Senior Lecturer in Biological Sciences, Faculty of Health and Social Care, University of the West of England, Bristol.

Alison Harris is Continence Nurse Specialist, Camden and Islington Community Healthcare Trust.

Dr Rachel Locke is Research Fellow, University of Sussex; and Liz Salter is Continence Adviser, Wiltshire and Swindon Healthcare NHS Trust, Swindon.

Lynn J Parker is Clinical Nurse Specialist, Infection Control, Sheffield's Teaching Hospitals NHS Trust, Northern General Hospital, Sheffield.

Ian Peate is Principal Lecturer, Adult Nursing and Health Care, University of Hertfordshire, Hatfield, Herts.

Patricia Penfold is Clinical Effectiveness Manager, Purey WST Nuffield Hospital, York.

Gary Porter-Jones is Respiratory Nurse, Ysbyty Gwynedd Hospital, Bangor, Gwynedd, North Wales.

Margaret Rew is Nurse Adviser, OPM Division, B.Braun Medical Ltd, Thorncliffe Park Estate, Sheffield.

Noreen Shields is Research and Development Officer for Women's Health, Greater Glasgow Health Board, Glasgow; Cathy Thomas was formerly Continence Facilitator, Greater Glasgow Community and Mental Health Services NHS Trust, Gartnaval Royal Hospital, Glasgow; Kate Benson is Physical Disability Leader, Glasgow Social Work Department, Glasgow; Kirsten Major is Health Economist, Ayrshire and Arran Health Board, Ayr; June Tree is Continence Manager, Greater Glasgow Community and Mental Health Services NHS Trust, Glasgow.

Elisabeth Stewart is Urology Nurse Practitioner, Surgical Nurse Specialist Department, Homerton NHS Trust, London.

Kate S Williams is Senior Research Fellow in the Department of Epidemiology and Public Health, Leicester University; R Phil Assassa is Consultant Obstetrician and Uro-gynaecologist at Pontefract General Infirmary; Nigel KG Smith is Consultant Geriatrician, Nottingham City Hospital Trust; Christine Shaw is Project Co-ordinator, Unit of Occupational and Health Psychology, Cardiff University.

Linda Winson is Continence Advisor, North East Wales NHS Trust, Connah's Quay, Flintshire.

Sue Woodward is Lecturer and Head of Section for Specialist and Palliative Care, Florence Nightingale School of Nursing and Midwifery, King's College, London.

Acknowledgements

We would like to express our appreciation to all the contributors involved in this book.

About the editors

Jeremy Pope Cruickshank MSc (Notts), BN (Hons), RGN, PGCE (FE) CMS, Dip PE is currently a Health Lecturer at the University of Nottingham, where he teaches on the Diploma in Nursing course and participates in the delivery of a variety of post-registration courses. A graduate of the Universities of Wales and Nottingham, he specialises in the acute areas of adult branch nursing. He has travelled to China, Australia, and the United States to witness first-hand the cultural differences in healthcare provision. His clinical background is in areas of high dependency/critical care and accident and emergency nursing. He is a member of the editorial boards of the *British Journal of Nursing* and Quay Books.

Sue Woodward RGN, MSc, PGCEA is currently Head of Specialist and Palliative Care at the Florence Nightingale School of Nursing and Midwifery, King's College, London. She teaches at pre-registration, post-registration and post-graduate levels and has responsibility for the delivery of specialist courses in neuroscience nursing and continence promotion. A graduate of the University of Surrey, with an MSc in Clinical Neuroscience, she is also the Programme Leader for critical care courses within her school. Her clinical background is in areas of neuroscience nursing and continence care. She is a member of the editorial boards of the *British Journal of Nursing* and the *International Journal of Nursing Studies*.

Introduction

Recently, in a series of publications, *Good Practice in Continence Services* (DoH, 2000), *The Essence of Care: Patient-focused benchmarking for health care practitioners* (DoH, 2001a) and the *National Service Framework for Older People* (DoH,2001b), the Department of Health (DoH) have been instrumental in strengthening the overall profile of continence services. Embodied within this guidance are strategies that recognise the importance of good practice and service provision within this expanding and innovative speciality. As Holmes (2001) succinctly comments 'continence care has finally come of age'.

One therapeutic intervention that exists from the range of options available in continence care is the practice of urethral catheterisation. Urinary catheter management is a crucial component of the nurse's role in both hospital and the community and although an extensively used clinical practice, it remains a skilled aseptic procedure. Necessitating an extensive understanding of the principles of patient assessment, catheter selection, infection control, drainage system management, effective interpersonal and teaching skills, it continues to demand a high degree of knowledge, robust training and competence.

Under the auspices of the Department of Health and the Wolfson Institute of Health Sciences (Thames Valley University) the EPIC Project has led to the development of *National evidence-based guidelines for preventing healthcare associated infections in England* (Pratt *et al*, 2001). Encompassed within this initiative are recommendations that re-enforce the principles of good practice in urethral catheter management. Divided into four distinct interventions of:

* assessing the need for catheterisation
* selection of catheter type
* aseptic catheter insertion
* catheter maintenance.

These evidence-based guidelines focus on the prevention of infections associated with indwelling urethral catheters (Pratt, 2000). When incorporated into local policy and procedure these guidelines can be suitably applied as a benchmark in the process of quality improvement and are available to facilitate the assessment of clinical effectiveness.

With such initiatives in place, this monograph, *Management of Continence and Urinary Catheter Care* is a judicious and significant addition to the existing literature on the subject. Written by experienced healthcare specialists with expertise in continence management it presents a selection of previously published peer-reviewed works from the *British Journal of Nursing*. The material, chosen for its quality and relevance, addresses the varied and interesting aspects of continence and urinary catheter care. The monograph has been organised into four sections:

1. Continence problems: Principles of assessment and management.
2. Catheterisation and catheter care: Evidence-based practice.
3. Minimising and troubleshooting common catheter problems.
4. Perspectives of education, research and audit.

This monograph is not intended to be presented as a definitive text on the speciality, rather a distillation of the knowledge and wide experience of the individual contributors. By drawing upon a number of recurring themes, the monograph aims to contribute to the exploration of current developments and applications in the topical field of urinary catheter management and seeks to represent the links between related theory and evidence-based practice. Written in a clear, focused and accessible style, augmented with illustrations, the monograph is designed to provide invaluable information for all members of the multi-professional team involved in the care of patients experiencing difficulties with continence.

In addition, it will be especially beneficial as a key source for all those involved in the process of benchmarking, especially when relating it to the core theme of continence, bladder and bowel care (DoH, 2001a). With its comprehensive referencing and helpful advice on the opportunities for further reading, it provides essential resource material, which will appeal particularly to pre-registration diploma and degree nursing students. It will also be a substantial aid for nurses undertaking in-service training or specialist post-registration programmes.

References

Department of Health (2000) *Good Practice in Continence Services*. The Stationery Office, London

Department of Health (2001a) *The Essence of Care: Patient-focused benchmarking for health care practitioners*. The Stationery Office, London

Department of Health (2001b) *National Service Framework for Older People*. The Stationery Office, London

Holmes J (2001) Continence care is not the weakest link. *Nurs Times* **97**(20): 53

Pratt RJ, Pellowe CM, Loveday HP *et al* (2000) *Epic Phase 1: The development of national evidence-based guidelines for preventing hospital-acquired infections in England associated with the use of short-term indwelling urethral catheters in acute care: Technical report 86*. Thames Valley University, London. www.epic.tvu.ac.uk

Pratt RJ, Pellowe CM, Loveday HP *et al* (2001) Guidelines for preventing infections associated with the insertion and maintenance of short-term indwelling urethral catheters in acute care. *J Hospit Infect* **47**(Suppl: Executive summary, S5–S9; Introduction, S13–S19; Guidelines, S39–S46)

Section one
Continence problems: Principles of assessment and management

1
Male patients with lower urinary tract symptoms 1: Assessment

Grace Dorey

Male lower urinary tract symptoms include frequency, nocturia, urgency, urge incontinence, stress incontinence, post-micturition dribble and post-prostatectomy incontinence. All of these symptoms can be treated conservatively. In this chapter, a detailed subjective and objective assessment is provided based on a Delphi study undertaken by the author. The objective assessment includes a digital rectal examination to assess the pelvic floor muscle strength in order to provide a patient-specific exercise programme. The diagnosis of stress incontinence, urge incontinence, post-prostatectomy incontinence, post-micturition dribble and functional incontinence is made from the assessment. Men with lower urinary tract symptoms need a detailed subjective and objective assessment before a diagnosis is made and individual treatment is planned.

Male lower urinary tract symptoms (LUTS) include nocturia, frequency, urgency, urge incontinence, stress incontinence, post-micturition dribble and post-prostatectomy incontinence (Neal, 1990; Hunter *et al*, 1996; de la Rosette *et al*, 1998). LUTS in men may be divided into bladder voiding and bladder filling symptoms (Abrams, 1994), as shown in *Table 1.1*.

Table 1.1: Bladder filling and voiding symptoms in men	
Filling symptoms	Frequency, urgency, urge incontinence, nocturia
Voiding symptoms	Hesitancy, poor stream, straining, incomplete emptying, intermittency, terminal dribble
Source: Abrams (1994)	

Moderate to severe LUTS occur in about 25–30% of men, aged 50 years and over, who have not undergone surgery and the prevalence increases with age (Garraway *et al*, 1991; Chute *et al*, 1993; Hunter *et al*, 1996). As far back as 1972, Milne *et al* noted that symptoms of urgency, frequency, and nocturia were present in 50% of American men, aged 62–90 years, who had not undergone surgery. The symptoms of bladder outlet obstruction, most commonly due to benign prostatic hyperplasia, were reported to affect one in three men over the age of 50 years in the UK (Garraway *et al*, 1991).

One of the most distressing LUTS is urinary incontinence. The prevalence of urinary incontinence in men increases with age and ranges from 3.6% in men aged 45 years to 28.2% in men aged 90 years or over (Thomas *et al*, 1980; Britton *et al*, 1990; Brocklehurst, 1993; Malmsten *et al*, 1997). The prevalence of reported urinary incontinence in men varies with the definition of incontinence (any leaking, damp pants, wet pants) and the threshold (number of leakage episodes) used.

The main causes of incontinence following transurethral resection of the prostate (TURP) or radical prostatectomy in preoperatively continent men are sphincter damage and detrusor dysfunction (Rudy *et al*, 1984; Emberton *et al*, 1996; Donnellan *et al*, 1997). A survey in England of 5276 patients who had undergone TURP found that one-third of men (n=1759 men) who were continent before surgery reported some incontinence three months post-prostatectomy (Emberton *et al*, 1996).

After radical prostatectomy, Donnellan *et al* (1997) reported that 6% of men were mildly incontinent, 6% were moderately incontinent and 4% were severely incontinent at one year after surgery. Koeman *et al* (1996) used a self-administered questionnaire in The Netherlands and reported that after radical prostatectomy nine out of 14 men had involuntary loss of urine at orgasm even though only one patient suffered from stress incontinence.

In order to ascertain the presence and extent of LUTS, a subjective and objective assessment needs to be undertaken by a nurse or physiotherapist. From this, a detailed diagnosis and treatment plan can be made. The plan may indicate the need for a referral from the nurse or physiotherapist to a urologist or GP, or it may reveal a treatment need. At discharge, the outcome measures may be compared with the detail elicited in the initial assessment.

The assessment described in this chapter is based on a consensus study using the Delphi technique (Dorey, 1999). The Delphi process took its name from the Oracle of Delphi's skills of interpretation and foresight (Sackman, 1975). The Delphi technique was designed by Helmer (1967) as a method of reaching consensus on any issue of importance. The main characteristics of the technique are anonymity, the administration of three rounds of questionnaires, or more if necessary, to individual experts, and feedback of the results from previous rounds to the participants (Pill, 1971; Linstone and Turoff, 1975; Chaney, 1987).

The Delphi technique has the advantage that all participants are able to express their views equally (Whitman, 1990). Conversely, Sackman (1975) argued that the Delphi technique failed to meet standards normally set for scientific studies in terms of reliability and validity. He argued that the method forced consensus and was weakened by not allowing participants to discuss issues. The 14 experts used in this study included physiotherapists, urology nurses, continence advisers, and urologists from five countries. They reached agreement after four rounds of questions and generated multiple data from expert consensus.

The experts generated detailed data concerning a classified system of male incontinence, subjective and objective assessments, treatment, advice and outcomes. All treatments should be preceded by a subjective assessment.

Subjective assessment

A subjective assessment is an assessment based on patient (subject) reported findings.

Patient details

Patient details should include the patient's age, occupation, hobbies and activities in order to make a lifestyle evaluation.

Main problem

It is necessary to have knowledge of the severity and duration of the main problem, the limitation of activities, quality of life and bothersome rating (0–10) caused by the main problem.

Symptoms

Questions may then be asked in order to evaluate the presenting symptoms of stress incontinence, urgency, and urge incontinence plus the factors provoking leakage (provocating factors), frequency, nocturia and nocturnal enuresis. In order to have knowledge of voiding (obstructive) symptoms, questions should be asked concerning: the flow rate; any difficulty starting voiding; any difficulty maintaining the stream; the strength of the stream; whether the voids are small; the presence of terminal dribble; and whether the bladder feels full after micturition. Patients should also be asked if they feel a sensation to void again on moving away from the bathroom, as this may indicate double-void instability (when a detrusor contraction causes leakage after micturition).

It is helpful to know if the patient has an awareness of leaking and a sensation of voiding. Does the patient have post-micturition dribble or constant dribble? Is it painful to pass urine and is the urine dark or smoky or does it contain blood? Any indication of pain in the pelvic area may be marked on a body chart.

Duration and severity of symptoms

The duration of each symptom needs to be noted and the improvement or deterioration to date recorded; the severity of each symptom can be marked on a visual analogue scale (0–10).

Amount of leakage

The amount of leakage may be ascertained from a description by the patient and may be described as a few drops, or a medium or large leakage, the number of pads used per day, their size and whether the pads are damp, wet, or soaked. Does the patient have an appliance and leg bag, use intermittent catheterisation or have an indwelling catheter?

Frequency of leakage

The frequency of leakage must be determined: is it daily, once a week, or once a month? When does the leakage occur? What are the leakage aggravators: are they coughing, sneezing, walking, moving, running water, caffeine, alcohol, medications, or some other trigger?

Urine stop test

Can the patient stop or slow down the flow of urine mid-stream? This question provides the opportunity to explain that this exercise can lead to retention of urine and therefore should not be practised.

Bowel activity

Does the patient suffer from constipation, straining to defecate, or practise digital evacuation? How many times a week does defecation occur? Are the faeces liquid, soft or firm? Is there faecal urgency, faecal incontinence, or incontinence of flatus? Does the patient use laxatives, and does he have a balanced diet?

Surgical history

It is necessary to know the dates and outcomes of TURP and any repeat TURPs, radical prostatectomy, the presence of a urethral stricture, and any other surgery.

Medical history

It is of interest to know if there are any family history trends. Has the patient suffered from prostatitis, how often, and was it acute or chronic? The symptoms of prostatitis may be malaise and fever in the acute stage before the onset of dysuria, urgency, frequency, and obstructive voiding.

In both the acute and chronic stages, there may be pelvic pain. Has he had acute or chronic cystitis and with how many episodes? Is he allergic to latex and therefore runs the risk of anaphylactic shock if the therapist uses latex gloves? Does he have any metal implants? This knowledge is necessary as it is a contraindication of electrical stimulation if there is metal in the treatment field. Does he smoke or have respiratory problems which makes stress incontinence leakage worse? Does he take anticholinergic medications, or alpha blockers, such as doxazosin (Cardura), to relax the bladder neck, 5-alpha-reductase inhibitors, such as finasteride (Proscar), to reduce prostate size; is he on antiandrogen treatment or take any other medication? What is the effect and side-effects of the medication? Has he undergone or is he undergoing radiotherapy? Is there a neurological problem such as diabetes, multiple sclerosis, Parkinson's disease, or a severe cervical or lumbar spine problem with neurological deficit?

Previous treatment

Has the patient had previous conservative treatment and what was the outcome?

Body mass index

What is the patient's height and weight, and what is his body mass index (BMI)? (Weight (kg) divided by height (m^2): BMI >30=obese).

Sexual problems

Does the patient have difficulty achieving or maintaining penile erection?

Functional factors

Is the patient able to stand for urination? Does he have adequate mobility and dexterity? Are there any environmental problems which make access to the bathroom difficult? Is he cognitively impaired or having psychological problems, and is there a patient support network?

Motivation

At this stage it is necessary to know if the patient has the ability and motivation to incorporate the therapy into his lifestyle in order to comply with an exercise programme or with lifestyle changes.

Investigations

It is essential to have the results of: (1) a urinalysis of mid-stream urine to eliminate urinary infection; (2) a uroflow, to monitor the force of the stream during micturition; and (3) a post-void residual examination, using ultrasound to the bladder, to eliminate retention of urine, before a clear diagnosis can take place. Other tests of interest are: (4) a blood test measuring the amount of prostate specific antigen (PSA) in men over 50 and under 75 years of age as an elevated PSA may be indicative of prostate cancer; (5) a rectal ultrasound scan to aid the diagnosis of prostatic cancer and benign prostatic hypertrophy; (6) uro-dynamics to diagnose genuine stress incontinence or detrusor instability and a low compliance bladder; and (7) flexible cystoscopy for the diagnosis of strictures and bladder tumours. A 24-hour pad test is useful before treatment and then at discharge as an outcome measure.

Frequency/volume chart

A frequency/volume chart (F/V) can provide detailed knowledge of the factors listed in *Table 1.2*. It aids the diagnosis between urge incontinence, usually with attendant frequency and nocturia, and stress incontinence.

Table 1.2: Information provided by a frequency/volume chart
Frequency of voiding
Maximum voided volume
Minimum voided volume
Amount of fluid intake
Amount of caffeine and alcohol intake
Amount of urinary output
Time of going to bed
Amount voided at night as polyuria is present if the amount voided at night is greater than 35% of the 24-hour volume (Weiss *et al*, 1998)
Frequency of leakage and the number of pads used per day

Objective assessment

An objective assessment is an assessment based on the findings seen by the therapist. The patient should be given the opportunity to be chaperoned either by a partner or friend or by a member of staff. The objective assessment should always begin with an explanation of the reasons for the need for a digital rectal examination (DRE). It should be explained that it is necessary to know that the muscles of the pelvic floor which control continence are working correctly.

The strength and endurance of these muscles can be best assessed by feeling them, the method of exercising can be checked and the correct amount of exercise given. The skin sensation can also be checked. If the patient is unhappy about a DRE, he may allow a perineal examination but he should not be persuaded against his wishes.

Following this detailed explanation, the patient must give informed consent to the objective examination and the consent must be entered in the patient notes. At this stage he should be given the opportunity to visit the lavatory. For the objective examination, the patient should be lying on his back with two pillows under his head with his knees bent and his feet on the plinth (crook lying position) without his underwear but with a sheet or paper sheet over his pelvis. He may retain his sheath and drainage system if he has one.

Abdominal examination

In the crook lying position the abdomen is palpated by the therapist wearing non-latex gloves for pain, masses that need referral, and bladder distension, which may indicate retention, or a hypotonic or atonic bladder. This may need training and practice under medical supervision. It may be possible to palpate a ridge marking the extent of a full, hard, bladder with retention. A hard swollen abdomen may indicate a bladder distended to the xiphisternum (the bone attached to the lower end of the sternum) and the need for immediate referral to a urologist.

Perineal examination

First it is necessary to observe the pelvic area in the crook lying position for congenital abnormalities such as hypospadias where the urethral meatus opens on the underside of the penis. At this stage, an enlarged testis, warts, haemorrhoids, and tumours may be identified. The skin condition should be examined for evidence of redness, infection, and excoriation in the penile, perineal, scrotal, and anal areas.

The patient may then be asked to tighten the anus as if to prevent wind escaping while the anal wink is observed. Then he can be asked to tighten at the front to prevent the flow of urine and feel a scrotal lift and the base of the penis pull back towards the abdomen. Following which, he is asked to give an unguarded cough which may provide evidence of leakage. He is then requested to cough while he is tightening his pelvic floor muscles at the front to prevent leakage; this may provide evidence of urinary control.

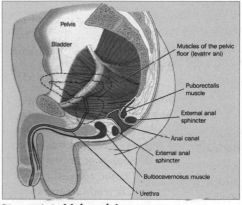

Figure 1.1: Male pelvic area

The S4 dermatome may be tested by using a cotton wool bud, or a gloved finger, by stroking gently either side of the perineum either side of the anus while asking the patient if it feels the same on both sides. If there is neurological deficit, S2 dermatome may be checked on the lateral surface of the buttock, lateral thigh, posterior calf and plantar heel and S3 dermatome may be checked on the upper two-thirds of the inner surface of the thigh. If neurological impairment is suspected, the bulbocavernosus reflex may be tested during the DRE. The patient should be prewarned. Gentle pressure on the glans penis during a digital rectal examination elicits an anal sphincter contraction unless there is neurological impairment.

Digital rectal examination

The therapist approximates a gloved index finger covered amply with lubricating gel to the anal meatus allowing the patient to feel the gel. The patient is then asked to bear down on to the finger as if he is letting wind escape. While the patient is bearing down, the finger is gently inserted straight, in a cephalad direction (towards the head) with the finger pad towards the coccyx. The finger can then be introduced to 1–2cm from the meatus and the integrity and tone of the external anal sphincter can be felt (Dixon *et al*, 1997). Any areas of pain should be noted.

With a lax sphincter, it may be possible to feel areas of scar tissue in the external anal sphincter where there is no muscle contraction. The patient should be asked to contract the anus and hold for five seconds, while the therapist grades the strength of the contraction and notes the duration of the hold. This can be repeated up to five times and then the ability to perform fast contractions noted. The examining finger can then be introduced to 3–4cm from the meatus and the anterior pull of puborectalis gently felt. This muscle is then graded, for any voluntary muscle in the body (0–5 for muscle strength), for the duration of the hold and for the ability to perform fast contractions. From this DRE, the anal sphincter and the puborectalis can then be assessed and recorded using the modified Oxford scale (Laycock, 1994) (*Table 1.3*).

Table 1.3: Assessment of strength of the pelvic floor muscles	
Grade	**Description**
0	Nil
1	Flicker
2	Weak
3	Moderate
4	Good
5	Strong
Source: Laycock (1994)	

Results of assessments

Following the subjective and objective assessment it is possible to make a problem list (multiple diagnoses), detail the aims of treatment, list the treatment modalities to be used, make a note of any advice to be given, and form a treatment plan.

Conclusion

A detailed subjective and objective assessment should be performed to provide a diagnosis of stress incontinence, urge incontinence, post-prostatectomy incontinence, post-micturition dribble, overflow incontinence, reflex incontinence, and functional incontinence. Patients can then receive the appropriate conservative treatment. *Chapter 2* will discuss the treatment of men with LUTS.

Key points

❖ The lower urinary tract symptoms in men of frequency, nocturia, urgency, urge incontinence, stress incontinence, post-micturition dribble and post-prostatectomy incontinence can be treated conservatively.

❖ The assessment has been compiled from the data generated by a Delphi study using 14 experts from five countries.

❖ The detailed subjective and objective assessment is necessary in order to make multiple diagnoses.

❖ Treatment progression is dependent on ongoing assessment.

References

Abrams P (1994) New words for old: lower urinary tract symptoms for 'prostatism'. *Br Med J* **308**: 929–30

Britton JP, Dowell AC, Whelan P (1990) Prevalence of urinary symptoms in men aged over 60. *Br J Urol* **66**: 175–6

Brocklehurst JC (1993) Urinary incontinence in the community — analysis of a MORI poll. *Br Med J* **306**: 832–4

Chaney H (1987) Needs assessment: a Delphi approach. *J Nurs Staff Devel* **3**: 48–53

Chute CG, Panser LA, Girman CJ, Oesterling JE, Guess HA, Jacobson SJ (1993) The prevalence of prostatism: a population-based survey of urinary symptoms. *J Urol* **150**: 85–9

de la Rosette JJMCH, Witjes WPJ, Schäfer W *et al* (1998) ICS-'BPH' study group: relationships between lower urinary tract symptoms and bladder outlet obstruction: results from the ICS-'BPH' study. *Neurourol Urodynam* **17**: 99–108

Dixon J, Dorey G, Eve B, Simonds K, Taylor V (1997) Post-prostatectomy incontinence. *J Assoc Chart Physiotherapist Women's Health* **80**: 35–8

Donnellan SM, Duncan HJ, MacGregor RJ, Russell JM (1997) Prospective assessment of incontinence after radical retropubic prostatectomy: objective and subjective analysis. *Urology* **49**(2): 225–30

Dorey G (1999) *Physiotherapy for the relief of male lower urinary tract symptoms: a Delphi study* (MSc thesis). University of East London

Emberton M, Neal DE, Black N *et al* (1996) The effect of prostatectomy on symptom severity and quality of life. *Br J Urol* **77**(2): 233–47

Garraway WM, Collins GN, Lee RJ (1991) High prevalence of benign prostatic hypertrophy in the community. *Lancet* **338**: 469–71

Helmer O (1967) *Analysis of the Future: The Delphi Technique*. Rand Corporation, Santa Monica

Hunter DJ, Berra-Unamuno A, Martin-Gordo A (1996) Prevalence of urinary symptoms and other urological conditions in Spanish men 50 years old or older. *J Urol* **155**(6): 1965–70

Koeman M, Van Driel MF, Weijmar Schultz WCM, Mensink HJA (1996) Orgasm after radical prostatectomy. *Br J Urol* **77**: 861–4

Laycock J (1994) Female pelvic floor assessment: the Laycock ring of continence. *J Nat Women's Health Group* (Australian Physiotherapy Association) **13**: 40–51

Linstone HA, Turoff M (1975) *The Delphi Method: Technique and Applications*. Addison-Wesley, Reading, Massachusetts

Malmsten UGH, Milsom I, Molander U, Norlen LJ (1997) Urinary incontinence and lower urinary tract symptoms: an epidemiological study of men aged 45 to 99 years. *J Urol* **158**: 1733–7

Milne JS, Williamson J, Maule MM (1972) Urinary symptoms in older people. *Mod Geriat* **2**: 198–212

Neal DE (1990) Prostatectomy — an open and closed case. *Br J Urol* **66**: 449–54

Pill J (1971) The Delphi method: substance, context, a critique and an annotated bibliography. *Socio-Econ Plann Sci* **5**: 57–71

Rudy DC, Woodside JR, Crawford ED (1984) Urodynamic evaluation of incontinence in patients undergoing modified Campbell radical retropubic prostatectomy: a prospective study. *J Urol* **132**: 708–12

Sackman H (1975) *A Delphi Critique*. Rand Corporation, Lexington Books, Lexington

Thomas TM, Plymat KR, Blannin J, Meade TW (1980) The prevalence of urinary incontinence. *Br Med J* **281**: 1243–5

Weiss JP, Stember DS, Blaivas JG, Brooks MM (1998) Nocturia in adults: classification and etiology. *Neurourol Urodynam* **17**: 467–72

Whitman I (1990) The committee meeting alternative: using the Delphi technique. *J Nurs Admin* **20**(7/8): 30–6

2

Male patients with lower urinary tract symptoms 2: Treatment

Grace Dorey

In *Chapter 1* the subjective and objective assessment of men with lower urinary tract symptoms (LUTS) was examined. This chapter will examine treatment protocols for stress incontinence, urge incontinence, post-prostatectomy incontinence, post-micturition dribble, overflow incontinence, reflex incontinence and functional incontinence. Pelvic floor muscle exercises, biofeedback, electrical stimulation, urge suppression techniques, and fluid intake are discussed. It is concluded that men with LUTS can benefit from conservative treatment.

Chapter 1 highlighted LUTS. Pelvic floor muscle exercises (PFMEs), biofeedback, bladder retraining, electrical stimulation, behavioural strategies and advice have all been utilised in the treatment of male LUTS. The benefits in men are not well researched; however, in non-randomised and non-controlled trials the results appear encouraging as discussed in detail in the literature review by Moore and Dorey (1999). Two of the three recent randomised, controlled trials (RCTs) support the intervention of physiotherapy treatment for men with LUTS (Paterson *et al*, 1997; Van Kampen *et al*, 1998; Moore *et al*, 1999).

The treatment options included in this chapter are based on a consensus study using the Delphi technique (Dorey, 1999). The Delphi process took its name from the Oracle of Delphi's skills of interpretation and foresight (Sackman, 1975). The Delphi technique was designed by Helmer (1967) as a method of reaching consensus on any issue of importance. The main characteristics of the technique are anonymity, the administration of three rounds of questionnaires, or more if necessary, to individual experts, and the feedback to the participants of the results from previous rounds (Pill, 1971; Linstone and Turoff, 1975; Chaney, 1987).

The Delphi technique has the advantage that all participants are able to express their views equally (Whitman, 1990). Conversely, Sackman (1975) argued that the Delphi technique failed to meet standards normally set for scientific studies in terms of reliability and validity. He argued that the method forced consensus and was weakened by not allowing participants to discuss issues. The 14 experts in this study included physiotherapists, urology nurses, continence advisers, and urologists from five countries. They reached agreement after four rounds of questions and generated multiple data from expert consensus.

Assessment

A detailed subjective and objective assessment will reveal the diagnosis or multiple diagnoses and must be undertaken before treatment is commenced (Dorey, 1999, 2000).

Treatment

Stress incontinence

Stress incontinence in men may occur as a result of sphincter damage following a prostatectomy (Donnellan *et al*, 1997). Physiotherapy incorporating PFMEs is potentially effective in alleviating stress incontinence caused by an incompetent urethral sphincter; this strategy is similar to that used in the treatment of women (Bø, 1995). Increased muscle work may increase blood flow to the capillary bed and therefore the passive mucosal seal (Dorey, 1999). PFMEs are non-invasive; they are not associated with serious complications and may be appropriate for patients with stress incontinence who wish to avoid surgery (Gray, 1992).

All treatments should start with patient education including an explanation of the patient's condition and the treatment options available. It is helpful to use a model of the male pelvis complete with musculature in order to explain the anatomy and physiology of the pelvic region (available from Educational and Scientific Products Ltd, Rustington, Sussex).

PFMEs for stress incontinence

PFMEs should be individually taught to make sure the patient is lifting up the pelvic floor and not bearing down as if defecating (ie, performing a Valsalva manoeuvre). Men can be encouraged to tighten and lift the pelvic floor muscles as in the control of flatus or when preventing the flow of urine and can practise in front of a mirror to observe a lift at the base of the penis and a scrotal lift (Paterson *et al*, 1997).

Men should be instructed to perform a penile lift by contracting the pelvic floor muscles, including the ischiocavernosus and bulbocavernosus muscles, and watch for a visible pull back of the base of the penis (Moore *et al*, 1999). Patients can be taught to palpate a contraction of the ischiocavernosus muscle at the perineum 2cm medially and 2cm anteriorly to the ischial tuberosity (*Figure 2.1*). The amount and progression of patient specific pelvic floor exercise is determined by individual assessment and digital rectal examination.

The convenient positions for practising PFMEs are in crook lying with the knees apart, standing with feet apart, and sitting with knees apart (Burgio *et al*, 1989; Paterson *et al*, 1997; Van Kampen *et al*, 1998; Moore *et al*, 1999). It is the intensity rather than frequency of work that is important and maximal voluntary effort causes muscle hypertrophy and increased muscle strength (Guyton, 1986;

Dinubile, 1991; Bø, 1995). In order to achieve full fitness, PFMEs should be taught for endurance as well as for muscle strength; this can be achieved by performing submaximal repetitive contractions (Guyton, 1986). Muscle training, therefore, depends on the motivation of the patient and the adherence to the pelvic floor exercise regimen (Jackson *et al*, 1996).

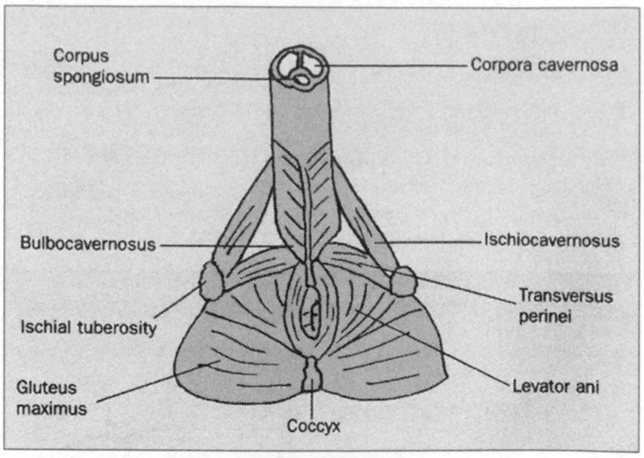

Figure 2.1: Male superficial perineal muscles

Home exercises

There is no evidence for an optimum number of repeat contractions. The quality of contraction is more important than the quantity. Exercises should be practised every day and include both fast and slow contractions. A typical programme practised twice a day may be: three maximal contractions in crook lying position, three maximal contractions in the sitting position, and three maximal contractions in the standing position. Contractions are held for the length of time in seconds determined at assessment and specific to the patient. Some contractions may be recruited quickly and some slowly. The patient can also be encouraged to lift the pelvic floor up 50% of their maximum while walking to encourage postural support. Men can be taught 'the knack' of tightening the pelvic floor muscles before activities which increase intra-abdominal pressure such as coughing, sneezing, rising from sitting, or lifting (Ashton-Miller and DeLancey, 1996).

Preoperative treatment

Before surgery, patients should receive education about the use of PFMEs, build up the strength and endurance of the pelvic floor muscles, and hopefully, in some cases, prevent or reduce incontinence. Sueppel (1998) realised the value of preoperative PFMEs and taught patients PFMEs before radical prostatectomy, with encouraging results.

Biofeedback for stress incontinence

Biofeedback is considered to make the patient more aware of pelvic floor muscle activity and encourage greater muscular effort (Burgio *et al*, 1989; Knight and Laycock, 1994; Jackson *et al*, 1996; Van Kampen *et al*, 1998). Biofeedback can be monitored by either manometric (pressure) recordings, using a rectal pressure probe, or by means of electromyography (EMG) using a rectal probe; alternatively surface sensors can be used to record the bioelectrical activity in the pelvic floor muscle.

One of the benefits of EMG is its use in functional positions. Two sticky sensors of small surface area may be placed longitudinally to the muscle monitored by EMG and may be placed over the coccyx and the perineal body. A third sensor is placed over a bony point, such as the patella, to act as a reference. There are, however, problems with EMG. Depending on the size of the sensor pad or probe used it may pick up electrical activity from the surrounding muscles. However, surface EMG is non-invasive, painless, and can also be used as an initiator of cerebral control, a tool of assessment, a motivator, and a method of recording; it can be used to both encourage and challenge the patient (Haslam, 1998). Many patients have no idea how to contract their pelvic floor and many do not understand the maximal effort needed. Biofeedback can often provide the necessary awareness for muscle re-education. Another adjunct to pelvic floor muscle re-education is the use of electrical stimulation.

Electrical stimulation for stress incontinence

There are two basic types of electrical stimulation which have been used on pelvic floor muscles: maximal electrical stimulation; and low intensity electrical stimulation.

Maximal electrical stimulation is applied pulsed at the maximum level tolerable for short periods of 20 minutes at a frequency of about 30Hz to produce a tetanic contraction and is used for stress incontinence (Jones, 1996). Low intensity electrical stimulation may be applied pulsed or continuous for several hours a day for several months. However, continuous low intensity electrical stimulation can lead to a conversion of muscle fibre type from fast twitch (type 2) to slow twitch (type 1) (Salmons and Henriksonn, 1981). This may produce an undesired effect as the recruitment of fast-twitch fibres of the pelvic floor muscles are necessary during rises in intra-abdominal pressure.

Table 2.1: Contraindications of electrical stimulation
Lack of consent
If the patient is anxious
Any broken skin in the area
Any metal in the field will concentrate the current and lead to a burn
Patients with severe cardiac problems and those with pacemakers
Cancer
Loss of sensation
Poor circulation

Electrical stimulation of the pelvic floor muscles may be delivered by rectal or surface electrodes. The rectal electrode contains positive and negative bands and is used alone. Surface electrodes may be placed on the coccyx and the perineum or on either side of the perineal body. Care should be taken to avoid burning that may occur with small electrodes. Contraindications to electrical stimulation are listed in *Table 2.1*.

A current of sufficient amplitude will excite nerve and muscle tissue in its field causing a muscular contraction. Electrical stimulation has been used for patients who are initially unable to contract the pelvic floor muscles. However, Berghmans *et al* (1998) noted that in five RCTs in women, electrical stimulation was found to be no more effective than PFMEs alone. In fact, Knight and Laycock (1998) found that pulsed, low intensity electrical stimulation may have a detrimental influence on female patients with genuine stress incontinence. In men, even less research has been conducted.

Electrical stimulation for stress urinary incontinence at a frequency of 30Hz or greater will produce a tetanic contraction with minimal risk of undue muscle fatigue, provided that the pulse train off-time is equal to or exceeds the on-time to prevent muscle fibre fatigue (Benton *et al*, 1981; Laycock *et al*, 1994). Knight and Laycock (1994) stated that a pulse width of 200 microseconds produces excitation at relatively low current intensity and is more comfortable than shorter pulse widths. They suggested that acute maximal electrical stimulation may benefit patients with very weak pelvic floor muscles. The real clinical benefit of electrical stimulation remains to be clarified. It may be that it can increase the circulation to the pelvic floor, or it may be useful to show patients how to contract the pelvic floor muscles.

Urge incontinence

The filling symptoms of frequency, nocturia, urgency, and urge incontinence can be treated with PFMEs, behavioural training, and lifestyle changes including fluid intake advice (Burgio *et al*, 1989; Paterson *et al*, 1997; Dorey, 1998; Van Kampen *et al*, 1998).

PFMEs for urge incontinence

PFMEs are used for urge incontinence to strengthen the pelvic floor musculature and regain the ability to control the urge to void urine. It is suggested that when the pelvic floor contracts the detrusor muscle will relax due to the perineopudendal facilitative reflex (Mahony *et al*, 1977).

Electrical stimulation for urge incontinence

Urge incontinence may be treated with continuous maximal biphasic electrical stimulation at a frequency of 5–10Hz for urge suppression, with a pulse width of 200 microseconds for up to 20 minutes (Fall and Lindstrom, 1991; Jones, 1994). Geirsson and Fall (1997) used stimulation parameters of 0.75milliseconds continuous biphasic waves with a frequency of 5Hz in the treatment of detrusor instability in order to cause reflex inhibition of detrusor contractions.

Lifestyle changes and behavioural techniques for urge incontinence

There are several non-invasive techniques which singly or combined may improve the symptoms of frequency, nocturia, urgency and urge incontinence. These include bladder retraining, the reduction of constipation, weight reduction, the adjustment of fluids, and the use of medications. In collaboration with other members of the healthcare team, bowel management, weight loss, medication review, and treatment of urinary tract infection may all improve symptoms. Patient education, attention to quantity, type and timing of fluid intake, avoiding constipation, and delaying the urge to micturate are now considered part of lifestyle changes which change previous behaviour patterns. Due to the limitations of current research, current knowledge and practice is based on opinion and consensus but not on strong evidence.

Bladder training for urge incontinence

Different names are given to urge suppression techniques known as bladder training. Bladder training (Frewen, 1979) may be referred to as bladder re-training (Mahady and Begg, 1981), bladder drill (Elder and Stephenson, 1980) or bladder re-education (Millard and Oldenburg, 1983) and is a method of consciously suppressing the urge to void in order to delay voiding and increase functional bladder capacity (Wells, 1988). Deferment techniques to delay voiding may be taught with strategies such as sitting on a hard chair, standing still, keeping calm, contracting the pelvic floor muscles and distraction (Laycock, 1995, personal communication). Patients undergoing bladder training need considerable encouragement, motivation, and determination to succeed.

Fluid intake

Guyton (1986) stated that normal fluid intake averages 2300ml per day, of which two-thirds (1518ml) is direct fluid and the remaining is a product of food synthesis. Weisberg (1982) found that a helpful gauge was 14–20ml of fluid intake per pound of body weight. It may be more helpful to monitor the 24-hour urine output, which should be between 1000 and 1500ml. However, normal intake should be increased during hot weather, with strenuous activity, and when eating salty foods. If the urine is dark, the patient should be encouraged to drink more fluid. Water is the best fluid to drink.

Diuretics

Natural diuretics are commonly xanthines, such as caffeine and theobromine, occurring primarily in beverages, which act chemically in the body to increase urine production. Caffeine occurs naturally in about 60 species of plants, most commonly coffee beans, tea leaves, cocoa seeds, and the cola nut (Moore, 1990). In 1988, Wells pointed out that caffeine is also added to several over-the-counter medications, commonly to counteract the drowsiness that the side-effect of the drug produces. Caffeine is a bladder irritant and stimulant with a diuretic effect. It can cause the smooth muscle of the detrusor muscle to contract with implications of nocturia, frequency, urgency, and urge incontinence (Addison, 1997). Addison considered that those men who are particularly at risk are those with detrusor instability, neurological disease, and elderly people. He stated caffeine should be reduced slowly in order to prevent withdrawal symptoms of headaches and drowsiness.

Cranberry juice

In the nineteenth century, North American Indians used crushed cranberries as a herbal remedy for the treatment of urinary tract infections (Bodel *et al*, 1959;

Moen, 1962). Although many studies have focused on the alteration in urinary pH (Fellers *et al*, 1933) or on increased hippuric acid levels (Bodel *et al*, 1959; Kinney and Blount, 1979), it is now believed that cranberry juice has a bacteriostatic effect by affecting the adherence of certain organisms to the bladder mucosa, in particular *Escherichia coli* (Beachy, 1981). Addison (1997) recommended cranberry juice for those patients with a high risk of urinary tract infection, those with cystitis from *E. coli*, patients with indwelling catheters, those undertaking intermittent self-catheterisation, or those using sheath drainage. He considered that the recommendation of cranberry juice should be supported by written patient information and be monitored and recorded with dosage, instructions, contraindications, side-effects, and expected outcomes.

There is controversy concerning the drinking of cranberry juice, as drinking in excess of one litre a day over a prolonged period may increase the risk of uric stone formation (Rogers, 1991). Other side-effects include gastritis and, for rheumatoid arthritis sufferers, increased joint pain (Addison, 1997). Diarrhoea is a side-effect in patients with irritable bowel syndrome (Leaver, 1996). For patients who simply do not like the taste, or find the juice too expensive, cranberry juice capsules can be purchased in health shops but there is no research on their comparison with cranberry juice (Leaver, 1996).

Medication for urge incontinence

It may be helpful for patients with severe urge incontinence and for patients with nocturnal enuresis to be prescribed anticholinergic medication while receiving conservative treatment. Oxybutynin or tolterodine may be prescribed by a GP. Side-effects include a dry mouth, drowsiness, and vision accommodation difficulties.

Post-prostatectomy incontinence

Post-prostatectomy incontinence should be treated according to the symptoms presented. Usually this is either stress incontinence or urge incontinence, but many patients may present with mixed incontinence.

Post-micturition dribble (PMD)

For patients suffering from PMD, a self-help technique called bulbar urethral massage or urethral milking can be used to ease this distressing condition. The patient is taught, after urinating, to place his fingers behind the scrotum and gently massage the bulbar urethra in a forwards and upwards direction in order to 'milk' the remaining urine from the urethra. It is helpful to use diagrams and models. Tightening the pelvic floor muscles before bulbar massage may help to prevent further leakage. Paterson *et al* (1997) undertook an interesting randomised single-blind trial to test the efficacy of urethral milking, but found PFMEs to be almost twice as effective as urethral milking and recommended PFMEs as a treatment for this condition. A 'squeeze out' contraction after urination will help to expel urine from the bulbar urethra.

Overflow incontinence

Self-intermittent catheterisation is used for patients with overflow incontinence due to an acontractile bladder or detrusor/sphincter dyssynergia. An acontractile bladder occurs when the smooth detrusor muscle fails to contract as a result of either lack of neurological control or overstretching. Detrusor/sphincter dyssynergia occurs when the detrusor muscle and sphincter contract simultaneously due to neurological impairment; this results in retention.

Reflex incontinence

Reflex incontinence is usually the result of a neurological condition. The bladder fills and empties automatically by an uncontrolled reflex contraction. The treatment for reflex incontinence consists of self-intermittent catheterisation, a sheath drainage system or, as a last resort, an indwelling catheter.

Functional incontinence

Functional incontinence is incontinence that is caused by problems of mobility and dexterity. Patients may find it difficult to reach the bathroom in time due to physical and environmental factors. Functional incontinence should be treated by improving the patient's environment, social care and aids, and lifestyle and clothing adaptations.

Further treatment

At the end of the treatment session, it is helpful to make a list of questions to ask the patient when he attends for his next treatment. The progression of the number and hold time of PFMEs will depend on the results of another rectal assessment to ascertain the strength and endurance of the pelvic floor muscles (Dorey, 2000).

Conclusion

Men with LUTS should be treated individually; subjective and objective assessment will indicate the specific treatment plan. Progression is dependent on ongoing assessment. For best practice, physiotherapists, continence advisers, urology nurses, urologists and GPs need to collaborate.

The challenge for professionals will be the integration of clinical evidence into practice and the promotion and implementation of prevention strategies. More research is needed to supplement these initiatives.

Consensus Statement, 1997

Key points

❖ A detailed subjective and objective assessment is necessary in order to make multiple diagnoses.

❖ In men, lower urinary tract symptoms (LUTS) of frequency, nocturia, urgency, urge incontinence, stress incontinence, post-micturition dribble, and post-prostatectomy incontinence can be treated conservatively.

❖ Treatment has been compiled from data supplied by a Delphi study using 14 experts from five countries.

❖ Treatment progression is dependent on ongoing assessment.

References

Addison R (1997) Cranberry juice: the story so far. *J Assoc Chart Physiother Women's Health* **80**: 21–2

Ashton-Miller JA, DeLancey JOL (1996) The Knack: use of precisely-timed pelvic muscle contraction can reduce leakage in SUI. *Neurourol Urodynam* **15**(4): 392–33

Beachy EH (1981) Bacterial adherence; adhesion receptor interactions mediating the attachment of bacteria to mucosal surfaces. *J Infect Dis* **143**: 325–45

Benton LA, Baker LL, Bowman BR, Waters RL, eds (1981) *Functional Stimulation: A Practical Clinical Guide.* Rancho Los Amigos Rehabilitation Engineering Centre, California: 1–78

Berghmans LCM, Hendriks HJM, Bø K *et al* (1998) Conservative treatment of stress urinary incontinence in women: a systematic review of randomised clinical trials. *Br J Urol* **82**: 181–91

Bø K (1995) Pelvic floor muscle exercise for the treatment of stress urinary incontinence: an exercise physiology perspective. *Int Urogynecology J* **6**: 282–91

Bodel PT, Cotran R, Kass EH (1959) Cranberry juice and antibacterial action of hippuric acid. *J Lab Clin Med* **54**(6): 881–8

Burgio KL, Stutzman RE, Engel BT (1989) Behavioral training for post-prostatectomy urinary incontinence. *J Urol* **141**: 303–6

Chaney H (1987) Needs assessment: a Delphi approach. *J Nurs Staff Devel* **3**: 48–53

Consensus Statement (1997) First International Conference for the Prevention of Incontinence, 25–27 June. The Continence Foundation, London

Dinubile NA (1991) Strength training. *Clin Sports Med* **10**(1): 33–62

Donnellan SM, Duncan HJ, MacGregor RJ, Russell JM (1997) Prospective assessment of incontinence after radical retropubic prostatectomy: objective and subjective analysis. *Urology* **49**(2): 225–30

Dorey G (1998) Physiotherapy for male continence problems. *Physiotherapy* **85**(11): 556–63

Dorey G (1999) *Physiotherapy for the relief of male lower urinary tract symptoms: a Delphi study* (MSc thesis). University of East London

Dorey G (2000) Male patients with lower urinary tract symptoms 1: Assessment. *Br J Nurs* **9**(8): 497–501

Elder DD, Stephenson TP (1980) An assessment of the Frewen regime in the treatment of detrusor dysfunction in females. *Br J Urol* **52**: 467–71

Fall M, Lindstrom S (1991) Electrical stimulation: a physiological approach to the treatment of urinary incontinence. *Urol Clin North Am* **18**(2): 393–407

Fellers CR, Redmon BC, Parrott RN (1933) Effect of cranberries on urinary acidity and blood alkali reserve. *J Nutr* **6**: 455

Frewen W (1979) Role of bladder training in the treatment of the unstable bladder in the female. *Urol Clin North Am* **6**: 273

Geirsson G, Fall M (1997) Maximal functional electrical stimulation in routine practice. *Neurourol Urodynam* **16**: 559–65

Gray M (1992) *Genitourinary Disorders.* Mosby Year Book, St Louis

Guyton AC (1986) *Textbook of Medical Physiology.* WB Saunders, Philadelphia

Haslam J (1998) Physiotherapy EMG/biofeedback. 2nd International Conference of the Association for Continence Advice: conference proceedings, Edinburgh

Helmer O (1967) *Analysis of the Future: The Delphi Technique.* Rand Corporation, Santa Monica

Jackson J, Emerson L, Johnston B, Wilson J, Morales A (1996) Biofeedback: a non-invasive treatment for incontinence after radical prostatectomy. *Urol Nurs* **16**(2): 50–4

Jones R (1994) Neuromuscular adaptability: therapeutic implications. *J Assoc Physiother Obstet Gynaecol* **75**: 12–7

Jones R (1996) Nerves, muscles and continence. *J Assoc Chart Physiother Women's Health* **79**: 3–6

Kinney AB, Blount M (1979) Effect of cranberry juice on urinary pH. *Nurs Res* **28**(5): 287–90

Knight SJ, Laycock J (1994) The role of biofeedback in pelvic floor re-education. *Physiotherapy* **80**: 145–8

Knight SJ, Laycock J (1998) Evaluation of neuromuscular electrical stimulation in the treatment of genuine stress incontinence. *Physiotherapy* **84**(2): 61–71

Laycock J, Plevnick S, Senn E (1994) Electrical stimulation. In: Schüssler B, Laycock J, Norton P, Stanton S, eds. *Pelvic Floor Re-education: Principles and Practice.* Springer-Verlag, London: 143–52

Leaver RB (1996) Cranberry juice. *Prof Nurse* **11**(8): 525–6

Linstone HA, Turoff M (1975) *The Delphi Method: Technique and Applications.* Addison-Wesley, Reading, Massachusetts

Mahady IW, Begg BM (1981) Long-term symptomatic and cystometric care of the urge incontinence syndrome using a technique of bladder re-education. *Br J Obstet Gynecol* **88**: 1038–43

Mahony DT, Laferte RO, Blais DJ (1977) Integral storage and voiding reflexes. *Neurology* **9**(1): 95–106

Millard RJ, Oldenburg BF (1983) The symptomatic, urodynamic and psychodynamic results of bladder re-education programs. *J Urol* **130**: 715–9

Moen DV (1962) Observations on the effectiveness of cranberry juice in urinary infections. *Wisconsin Med J* **61**: 282–3

Moore H (1990) Caffeine. *Which?* June: 314–17

Moore KN, Dorey G (1999) Conservative treatment of urinary incontinence in men: a review of the literature. *Physiotherapy* **85**(2): 77–87

Moore KN, Griffiths DJ, Hughton A (1999) A randomised controlled trial comparing pelvic muscle exercises with pelvic muscle exercises plus electrical stimulation for the treatment of post-prostatectomy urinary incontinence. *Br J Urol* **83**: 57–65

Paterson J, Pinnock CB, Marshall VR (1997) Pelvic floor exercises as a treatment for post-micturition dribble. *Br J Urol* **79**: 892–7

Pill J (1971) The Delphi method: substance, context, a critique and an annotated bibliography. *Socio-Econ Plan Sci* **5**: 57–71

Rogers J (1991) Pass the cranberry juice. *Nurs Times* **87**(48): 36–7

Sackman H (1975) *A Delphi Critique.* Rand Corporation, Lexington Books, Lexington

Salmons S, Henriksonn J (1981) The adaptive response of skeletal muscle to increased use. *Muscle Nerve* **4**: 94–105

Sueppel C (1998) Timing of pelvic floor muscle strengthening exercises and return of continence in post-prostatectomy patients. Conference proceedings of the Society of Urologic Nurses and Associates, 4th National Multi-Specialty Nursing Conference on Urinary Continence, Florida

Van Kampen M, De Weerdt W, Claes H *et al* (1998) *Contribution of pelvic floor muscle exercises in the treatment of impotence* (PhD thesis). Katholieke Universiteit Leuven, Belgium

Weisberg HF (1982) *Water, Electrolyte and Acid-base Balance.* 2nd edn. Williams and Wilkins, Baltimore

Wells TJ (1988) Additional treatments for urinary incontinence. *Topics Geriat Rehab* **3**(2): 48–57

Whitman I (1990) The committee meeting alternative: using the Delphi technique. *J Nurs Admin* **20**(7/8): 30–6

3

Nocturia, nocturnal polyuria and secondary nocturnal voiding

Ray Addison

Getting up once to the toilet at night is normal. Getting up more than once may be abnormal. Potential causes include: nocturia, which is bladder related; nocturnal polyuria, which is cardiac in origin; and being awake for a variety of reasons that are not linked to the bladder. Bladder problems, therefore, are not always the reason for frequency in micturition at night and treatment will only be effective if the correct cause and/or causes are identified. The most useful investigation to help with diagnosis is a frequency volume chart linked to an assessment identifying causes of secondary nocturnal voiding and nocturnal polyuria. Getting up to the toilet at night will not always be successfully treated by anticholinergics. Charting is the key to diagnosis, appropriate interventions and successful outcomes. This chapter will focus on working definitions, prevalence, causes, investigations and treatment options for nocturia, nocturnal polyuria and secondary nocturnal voiding.

It is important that nurses and other healthcare practitioners understand the definitions of nocturia, nocturnal polyuria and secondary nocturnal voiding as the interventions are not always related to the bladder alone (*Table 3.1*).

Table 3.1. Definitions of nocturia, nocturnal polyuria and secondary nocturnal voiding
Nocturia: commonly defined as awakening from sleep because of the desire to void (Shah, 1994; Stephenson and Mundy, 1994; Winder, 1996; Abrams, 1997; Getliffe and Dolman, 1997; Khullar, 1997; Bhatti and Watson, 1998; Weiss *et al*, 1998)
Nocturnal polyuria: where large volumes of urine are passed at night, greater than 33% of the total daily volume (Weiss *et al*, 1997; Drake *et al*, 1998; Weiss *et al*, 1998)
Secondary nocturnal voiding: voiding that is the result of being awake and therefore is not true nocturia (Drake *et al*, 1998)

Normal voiding

Sometimes nocturia can be classed as normal (Getliffe and Dolman, 1997). Millard (1996) states that 33% of the population get up once during the night. Winder (1996) regards twice or more episodes of nocturia as abnormal. Drake *et al* (1998) estimate that 80% of the male population will get nocturia in later life and Weiss *et al* (1998) consider that males are more likely to have nocturnal polyuria than females. Wise (1997) believes that almost 70% of nocturia is caused by detrusor instability.

There is a strong relationship between the prevalence of nocturia and increasing age (Stewart *et al*, 1992; Stephenson and Munday, 1994; Millard, 1996; Winder, 1996; Abrams, 1997; Khullar, 1997; Bhatti and Watson, 1998; Drake *et al*, 1998; Rembratt and Mattiasson, 1998; Weiss *et al*, 1998). Weiss *et al* (1998) found that 72% of people over 65 get up once at night and 24% routinely rise three or more times. It is estimated that at the age of 60 most people get up once; this rises to twice at the age of 70, three times at 80 and four times at 90 (Stephenson and Mundy, 1994; Khullar, 1997; Wise, 1997).

An American retrospective study looked at the medical records of 194 patients (Weiss *et al*, 1997). It found that 5% had nocturnal polyuria, 57% had detrusor instability (overactive bladder) and 36% had polyuria with detrusor instability. It concluded that 43% of patients reviewed had over-production of urine at night and that the problem was multifactorial.

The effects of nocturia can be very distressing. People commonly suffer from fatigue due to sleep deprivation (Weiss *et al*, 1998). In addition, it has been found that falls are more common among elderly people with nocturia (Stewart *et al*, 1992).

Causes

Nocturia

There are many causes of nocturia. It may be due to an obstruction such as an enlarged prostate in men which causes a voiding problem (Shah, 1994; Millard, 1996; Winder, 1996; Bhatti and Watson, 1998; Drake *et al*, 1998). Neurological disease can also cause detrusor instability resulting in nocturia (Rushton, 1997; Drake *et al*, 1998). Nocturia is likely to be a symptom in people with idiopathic detrusor instability (Abrams, 1997; Wise, 1997; Bhatti and Watson, 1998; Drake *et al*, 1998). A small bladder capacity combined with a non-compliant bladder will also increase the risk of nocturia (Millard, 1996; Abrams, 1997). Nocturia is more common in pregnancy (Bhatti and Watson, 1998).

Nocturia can also be caused by irritative or inflammatory conditions of the bladder, eg. infection and cystitis (Dahistrand *et al*, 1996; Bhatti and Watson, 1998; Drake *et al*, 1998), bladder cancers (Abrams, 1997; Wise, 1997; Bhatti and Watson, 1998; Drake *et al*, 1998), stones (Bhatti and Watson, 1998; Drake *et al*, 1998), and medications which have nocturia as a side-effect (Bhatti and Watson, 1998; Drake *et al*, 1998).

Nocturnal polyuria

Nocturnal polyuria can occur for a variety of reasons. If more than one factor is involved then the situation becomes more complex. Excessive evening fluid intake relates to increased output during the night (Shah, 1994; Millard, 1996; Bhatti and

Watson, 1998; Drake *et al*, 1998) and cardiac failure can cause increased urinary output due to improved venous return to the heart during sleep (Saito *et al*, 1993; Shah, 1994; Abrams, 1997; Bhatti and Watson, 1998; Drake *et al*, 1998).

People with postural oedema will find that elevating their legs in bed improves circulation and increases urinary output (Millard, 1996; Abrams, 1997; Khullar, 1997). This increased urinary output at night may also be enhanced by a lack of diurnal hormone control due to a reduction in the production and influence of the antidiuretic hormone which reduces urine production at night (Asplund and Aberg, 1991; Saito *et al*, 1993; Millard, 1996; Abrams, 1997; Bhatti and Watson, 1998).

Other causes of nocturnal polyuria include: renal failure (Bhatti and Watson, 1998; Drake *et al*, 1998); hypertension (Drake *et al*, 1998); medication, such as long-acting diuretics (Drake *et al*, 1998); diabetes (Bhatti and Watson, 1998); hypercalcaemia (Bhatti and Watson, 1998; Drake *et al*, 1998); hypo-albuminaemia (Bhatti and Watson, 1998); and peripheral vascular disease (Bhatti and Watson, 1998).

Secondary nocturnal voiding

Secondary nocturnal voiding also has a number of possible causes. Insomnia is by far the most recognised cause of secondary nocturnal voiding (Shah, 1994; Winder, 1996; Abrams, 1997; Benness and Hill, 1997; Bhatti and Watson, 1998; Drake *et al*, 1998) and, when the patient has become conditioned to wake at night due to established behaviour patterns, habit is another cause (Millard, 1996; Abrams, 1997). Disturbed sleep can be the result of pain (Abrams, 1997; Bhatti and Watson, 1998; Drake *et al*, 1998), sleep apnoea (Dahistrand *et al*, 1996; Bhatti and Watson 1998; Drake *et al*, 1998) and depression (Bhatti and Watson, 1998).

Assessment

Most patients suffering from nocturia, nocturnal polyuria and secondary nocturnal voiding are referred to a urologist (Weiss *et al*, 1998). It must be remembered that people can have all three conditions at the same time and this must be identified in the assessment process. For example, a patient may present with nocturia as a result of prostatic enlargement but may also suffer from insomnia which causes a secondary nocturnal voiding problem. In this situation, a prostatectomy will not solve the nocturia.

Another patient presenting with nocturia may be treated with anticholinergics (drugs used to treat detrusor instability); however, if this patient has nocturnal polyuria and gets up at night because his bladder is at capacity, diuretic therapy is needed to resolve the situation. To be most effective, diuretics are best taken at midday.

Therefore, some patients may need a double or triple therapy approach if they have a combination of nocturia, nocturnal polyuria and secondary nocturnal voiding problems.

Investigations

The four main investigations for nocturia are listed in *Table 3.2*. Bhatti and Watson (1998) and Drake *et al* (1998) also recommend using a prostate screening questionnaire and taking a history, blood chemistry and urinalysis. Bhatti and Watson (1998) go further and indicate that an abdominal X-ray and a physical examination are required.

Table 3.2: Main investigations for nocturia
A frequency, volume and intake chart (Millard, 1996; Abrams, 1997; Weiss *et al*, 1997; Bhatti and Watson, 1998; Drake *et al*, 1998; Weiss *et al*, 1998). This is the most common investigation
Urodynamic studies in selected patients (Shah, 1994; Weiss *et al*, 1997; Bhatti and Watson, 1998; Drake *et al*, 1998; Weiss *et al*, 1998)
A post-void ultrasound which may indicate a voiding problem by identifying residual urine (Weiss *et al*, 1997; Bhatti and Watson, 1998; Weiss *et al*, 1998)
Urine flow rate may show some form of outflow obstruction or degree of detrusor failure where the bladder muscle is unable to contract to expel urine effectively (Millard, 1996; Bhatti and Watson, 1998; Drake *et al*, 1998)

Treatment

In the treatment of nocturia, nocturnal polyuria and secondary nocturnal voiding, it is helpful to divide up the treatment categories as indicated in *Table 3.3*.

Table 3.3: Treatment categories
Nocturnal polyuria
Nocturia with physical outflow obstruction
Nocturia due to detrusor instability with no outflow obstruction
Nocturia with neurological outflow obstruction
Secondary nocturnal voiding
Inflammatory or irritative conditions to the urinary tract

Nocturnal polyuria

In the treatment of nocturnal polyuria it is important to restrict fluid intake (Millard, 1996; Abrams, 1997; Bhatti and Watson, 1998), reducing the total fluid intake to about 1.5 litres per day. Evening fluid restriction may be a useful strategy as well as discouraging drinking during the night. A review of the patient's fluid preferences may reveal alcohol and caffeine consumption which can aggravate the problem by reducing the depth and length of sleep as well as acting as a diuretic (Millard, 1996; Bhatti and Watson, 1998). Millard (1996) advises a reduction in salt intake as this will affect fluid balance. Millard (1996) and Abrams (1997) both advise the elevation of legs during the day to reduce postural oedema. Weiss *et al* (1998) suggest that compressive stockings may also help with postural oedema and venous return.

Bhatti and Watson (1998) suggest that the patient's medication should be reviewed. Taking a diuretic during the day may reduce the volume of urine produced at night, thus giving therapuetic benefits (Millard, 1996; Abrams, 1997; Bhatti and Watson, 1998; Weiss *et al*, 1998). Desmopressin is also considered useful for nocturia because of its antidiuretic effects although it is currently only licensed for use in people with multiple sclerosis under 60 years of age and in the treatment of diabetes insipidus and bleeding oesophageal varices (Shah, 1994; Abrams, 1997; Wise, 1997).

Nocturia caused by physical obstruction

In men with an enlarged prostate and associated voiding problems, surgery may be necessary (Bhatti and Watson, 1998). Medication, such as finasteride, is now available to shrink the prostate and this may reduce the patient's symptoms of nocturia. An indwelling Foley catheter can be used in patients awaiting surgery or those not fit for surgery who have a considerable residual urine (over 300ml), and/or kidney complications and/or symptoms which are bothersome, such as urgency and nocturia.

Treatment of nocturia caused by detrusor instability

There are two main ways of treating nocturia caused by detrusor instability. Millard (1996) recommends bladder retraining with the aim of increasing bladder capacity and the intervoiding period. Bhatti and Watson (1998) recommend drug therapy in the form of oxybutynin; this is an anticholinergic which increases bladder capacity by diminishing unstable detrusor contractions. Wise (1997) suggests that imipramine has the same action. Other drugs have also been developed and are available within the UK.

Often bladder retraining can be combined with anticholinergic drug therapy to give symptom relief as medication should not be viewed as a life-long solution. Bhatti and Watson (1998) also consider cystodistension, ie. bladder expansion by mechanical means, under anaesthetic as a treatment option.

Nocturia caused by neurological obstruction

In patients with neurological disease, bladder dysfunction is common. For example, voiding dysfunction is common in multiple sclerosis. Available treatment options include: vibration to the lower abdominal wall to initiate detrusor contractions and voiding; intermittent self-catheterisation; an indwelling long-term catheter; or surgery to the bladder to enlarge (ileo-cystoplasty) or divert it (ileal conduit) (Kirby, 1996).

Secondary nocturnal voiding

There are many reasons why patients suffer from secondary nocturnal voiding which are too numerous to explore within the scope of this chapter. However, an example from the author's clinic is of a man who's nocturia was dramatically improved after being given analgesia for his arthritic hand. It is important for the healthcare professional to be aware of possible causes in order to assess, investigate and plan and initiate appropriate care. Evaluation is important to see if the interventions have improved sleep and the symptoms.

Inflammatory or irritative conditions to the urinary tract

The results of urinalysis will reveal, along with the symptoms, eg. burning pain, frequency, nocturia and bleeding, whether infection is present. Treating a urinary tract infection may be therapeutic in reducing nocturia. Increasing fluids for a urinary tract infection is standard practice but these should be reduced once the symptoms have gone and the urine is clear. Caffeine and alcohol are irritant substances and it is worth experimenting with withdrawal to see if they are irritant to the patient. Bladder stones and radiotherapy to the pelvic area are also causes of inflammation and irritation.

Conclusion

Millard (1996) states that patients may have to accept that nocturia and nocturnal polyuria are a permanent part of their lives. Nocturia has been described as a common problem and age plays an important part in the increase of its incidence. It is bothersome as sleep is disturbed. As the causes are often multifactorial a double or triple approach to therapy is required.

Health education material is required to help patients deal appropriately with their problems. A frequency volume and intake chart should be used which is specifically designed to highlight nocturia, nocturnal polyuria and secondary nocturnal voiding as this will aid professionals in appropriate interventions.

Key points

❖ Nocturia is a common problem that increases with age and which may become bothersome.

❖ Nocturia is a multifactorial problem, not always related to the bladder.

❖ Assessment and investigations must aim to identify true nocturia, nocturnal polyuria and secondary nocturnal voiding.

❖ A triple therapy approach is recommended, related to cause and symptoms.

❖ A well designed chart is the best investigatory tool to identify the true cause of nocturia.

References

Abrams P (1997) *Urodynamics.* 2nd edn. Springer-Verlag, London

Asplund R, Aberg H (1991) Diurnal variation in the levels of antidiuretic hormone in the elderly. *J Int Med* **229**: 135–41

Benness C, Hill S (1997) Frequency, urgency and painful bladder syndromes. In: Cardozo IJ, ed. *Urogynecology.* Churchill Livingstone, Edinburgh: 359

Bhatti A, Watson G (1998) Nocturia. *Urology News* **2**(4): 15

Dahistrand C, Hedner J, Wang YH *et al* (1996) Snoring: a common cause of voiding disturbance in elderly men. *Lancet* **347**: 270–1

Drake MJ, Mills IW, Noble JG (1998) *The diverse causes of nocturia in men.* Abstracts of the 28th meeting of the International Continence Society, Jerusalem. Abstract **290**: 276–7

Getliffe K, Dolman M (1997) *Promoting Continence: A Clinical and Research Resource.* Baillière Tindall, London

Khullar V (1997) History and examination. In: Cardozo L, ed. *Urogynecology.* Churchill Livingstone, Edinburgh: 88

Kirby RS (1996) *Patient Pictures — Urological Surgery.* Health Press, Oxford

Millard RJ (1996) *Bladder Control: A Simple Self-Help Guide.* Maclennan and Petty, Sydney

Rembratt A, Mattiasson A (1998) *The prevalence of nocturia in the general population.* Abstracts of the 28th meeting of the International Continence Society, Jerusalem. Abstract **241**: 201–2

Rushton D (1997) Neurological disorders. In: Cardozo L, ed. *Urogynecology.* Churchill Livingstone, Edinburgh: 497

Saito M, Kondo A, Kato T *et al* (1993) Frequency volume charts: comparison of frequency between elderly and adult patients. *Br J Urol* **72**: 38–41

Shah PJR (1994) The assessment of patients with a view to urodynamics. In: Mundy AR, Stephenson TP, Wein AJ, eds. *Urodynamics.* Churchill Livingstone, Edinburgh: 88

Stephenson TP, Mundy AR (1994) The urge syndrome. In: Mundy AR, Stephenson TP, Wein AJ, eds. *Urodynamics.* Churchill Livingstone, Edinburgh: 265

Stewart RB, Moore MT, May FE *et al* (1992) Nocturia: a risk factor for falls in the elderly. *J Am Geriatr Soc* **40**: 1217–20

Weiss JP, Stember DS, Blaivis JG (1997) Nocturia in adults: classification and etiology. *Neurourol Urodynamics* **16**(5): 401

Weiss JP, Blaivis JG, Stember DS *et al* (1998) Nocturia in adults: etiology and classification. *Neurourol Urodynamics* **17**(5): 467–72

Winder A (1996) Assessment and investigation of urinary incontinence. In: Norton C, ed. *Nursing for Continence.* Beaconsfield Publishers, Beaconsfield: 37–40

Wise B (1997) Detrusor instability and hyperreflexia. In: Cardozo L, ed. *Urogynecology.* Churchill Livingstone, Edinburgh: 295

4

Impact of urinary incontinence on the quality of life of women

Alison Harris

There is a lot of debate among continence specialists as to the impact that urinary incontinence (UI) has upon the sufferer's quality of life (QoL). Furthermore, healthcare professionals involved in delivering care are examining ways to measure the outcomes of their healthcare interventions, in terms of not only symptom relief, but also patient-specified improvements to QoL. Healthcare professionals have yet to agree upon one standard tool for measuring the effect of UI upon sufferers' QoL. This chapter examines some of the current research on UI as experienced by females living in their own homes and its impact on their QoL.

Healthcare professionals who have developed an interest in continence (ie. nurses, doctors, physiotherapists) recognise that urinary incontinence (UI) can bring about changes in the individual's lifestyle in relation to social interactions, sexuality, career and sense of physical well-being (Kelleher *et al*, 1995). Approximately 5% of the UK population experience incontinence at least twice a month (Norton, 1996). Driven by the increasing expenditure on incontinence products and devices (£56 million in 1991) (Norton, 1996), most health authorities now employ a continence adviser.

The definition of UI as set out by the International Continence Society is:

The involuntary loss of urine which is objectively demonstrable and a social or hygiene problem

cited in Norton, 1996

Many of the research studies (Ashworth and Hagan, 1993; Norton *et al*, 1988) state that there is no commonly accepted definition whereby UI can be consistently measured along a continuum from minimum to severe. Thus, healthcare professionals are learning to recognise that UI symptoms are as severe as the sufferer says they are and that any attempt to define degrees of severity is to risk misinterpreting how UI affects the individual.

Bech (1993) states:

Health-related quality of life is what the patient himself feels is an improvement globally, the incremental validity of health. It is a subjective, psychological dimension.

The use of quality of life measures should allow healthcare professionals to evaluate the outcomes of their interventions in terms of holistic, patient-centred needs as well as helping them to understand the impact of deviations from patient well-being and the reasons why people present for treatment. The problem for the healthcare professional is in finding a well validated and reliable tool that measures the subjective phenomena of QoL and how it is affected by UI.

Glossary
Detrusor instability or an overactive bladder: a condition characterised by involuntary bladder contractions or pressure rises during bladder filling.
Frequency: voiding more than the considered normal per day, often quoted as more than ten times a day.
Neurogenic bladder: one that does not produce an effective voiding contraction due to nerve damage of the bladder or lower spinal cord.
Oxybutynin: an anticholinergic drug that is used predominantly in the treatment of detrusor instability to reduce frequency and increase the bladder holding capacity by sedating the bladder or detrusor muscle.
Stress incontinence: is caused by a failure to hold urine during bladder filling, in the absence of a detrusor contraction, as a result of an incompetent urethral sphincter mechanism.
Urge incontinence: involuntary loss of urine as a result of a detrusor contraction.

As a continence nurse specialist working in a modern healthcare system, the author has both an employer's expectation and a professional interest in ensuring that the clinical effectiveness of the care given is evaluated. Nurses have long understood that health is a balance of 'social and personal resources as well as physical capabilities' (World Health Organization, 1984) and thus effectiveness of care must be measured not only quantitatively, eg. by monitoring the reduction in symptoms experienced, but also through studying how healthcare interventions affect the holistic quality of patients' lives.

There is a richness of data available on measuring QoL but few of the researchers have acknowledged whether they extended their findings into practice. This chapter will explore the ways in which the findings from existing QoL research can be applied to practice in caring and treating those individuals with Ul.

The relationship between urinary incontinence and quality of life

The relationship between QoL and UI is a complex one and many researchers, while trying to quantify a phenomenon that is by nature qualitative, may have over simplified the experience of incontinence sufferers. While an assumption can be made that there will be a correlation between QoL and UI, it may be that it is not a strong one.

The other problem of creating a tool to objectively measure an individual's QoL is that the creator of the tool may impose many of his/her own assumptions.

The challenge for the researcher is to demonstrate the consistency of the tool's findings, thereby illustrating its validity and reliability. The tool's usability is also important to practitioners working in today's health service.

It is recognised that approximately 10% of incontinent people are known to the health and social services (Norton, 1996). Many of the research studies carried out on QoL measures were undertaken by physicians and surgeons within outpatient clinics, using a purposive sample of individuals voluntarily presenting for treatment (Norton *et al*, 1988; Fonda *et al*, 1995). Therefore, these samples may not be representative of the total incontinent population who, as shall be discussed later, are often too embarrassed or lack the motivation to seek help, especially from doctors (Norton *et al*, 1988; Ashworth and Hagan, 1993). This may give bias to some of the research findings.

A qualitative study by psychologists (Ashworth and Hagan, 1993) reported on the coping mechanisms employed by UI sufferers which included not recognising themselves as incontinent and concealing their problem.

A paradigm of urinary incontinence

Norton *et al* (1988) conducted a quantitative study of 201 women over the age of 16 in a purposive sample taken from women attending a urodynamic clinic. The aim of the study was to examine the reasons why women with UI delayed seeking help. Norton *et al* (1988) found that women over 65-years old were twice as likely as women under 35 to delay seeking help for their incontinence. The older women's reasons were embarrassment at seeking help from their GP and fear of surgery.

Gallagher (1998) analysed 17 women living at home who experienced UI at least once a week. All of the sample were over 60 years old, but the highest number, 40%, were between 81 and 83 years. The validity of Gallagher's study is reduced by the small sample; however, it was noted by the author that the study could be used as a pilot and it does add a nursing dimension to a largely medical field of study. Gallagher found that while there was a significant, negative correlation between UI and physical activity, social relationships and travel, there was not a significant relationship between UI and emotional health (eg. anxiety, depression and embarrassment). Gallagher's findings led her to suppose that elderly females may normalise UI as part of the ageing process.

For Norton *et al*'s (1988) and Gallagher's (1998) findings to be meaningful to healthcare practice, more understanding is required of what UI means to different age groups, which urinary symptoms are considered tolerable and what it is that eventually causes individuals to seek help.

The stigma of UI is a recurrent finding in the literature (Norton *et al*, 1988; Ashworth and Hagan, 1993; Grimby *et al*, 1993). Ashworth and Hagan (1993) used a qualitative approach to examine the reasons why 28 women, ranging from 25–55 years old, were self-managing their incontinence. The sample comprised volunteers obtained using a newspaper advertisement which makes an examination of the sample difficult as they could be regarded as cooperative and forthcoming individuals who do not display some of the embarrassment and reserve of many incontinent sufferers. Their reasons for responding were not clarified by the author.

Ashworth and Hagan used an unstructured interview that was conducted in the individual's own home as the authors felt this would 'give sufferers a voice'. The respondents believed that UI was often associated with elderly and demented women and the stigma of UI prevented younger women coming forward for help. The taboo nature of incontinence prevented discussion of problems in a social setting and thus the sufferers were not optimising their potential for self-help. This qualitative approach gives a more descriptive picture than some of the quantitative studies and, within the relatively small sample, generates themes that could be further developed by a larger sample (eg. the development of a terminology that is acceptable to sufferers for the discussion of their problems or the feelings of loss aroused by UI).

Ashworth and Hagan (1993) found that incontinence was not viewed as a legitimate medical problem, possibly another reason why people with UI do not present for help. This is echoed in a pilot study undertaken by Smith (1998) which examined the attitudes of health workers to UI in elderly people. A mailed questionnaire, drawn up by a multidisciplinary group and piloted to minimise ambiguity and maximise response rate, was sent to a randomly selected sample of 200, equally divided between GPs, hospital doctors, practice nurses and nursing home nurses. The pre-determined response rate of 40% was met with a return of 46.5%. Nurses had the highest return rate and Smith (1998) recognised that this could imply that they had a greater interest in the subject and that the study might need repeating with a larger sample size to enhance the reliability of the data.

The analysis of the data showed that GPs exhibited the least healthy attitude towards the individual assessment of continence in elderly people. UI in the elderly is often treatable, but requires individual assessment and management. The implications for practice of these combined factors, with GPs often being the first point of call for UI sufferers, is that an increasing number of women may advance into very old age with UI that has not received the appropriate treatment. This in turn has implications for the growing cost of health care.

Chiverton *et al* (1996), in a joint nursing and medical quantitative study, examined the correlation between mastery over one's life (ie. feeling able to control events) and depression, and/or self-esteem and depression, in women with UI and the impact of these dependent variables on QoL. Chiverton *et al* (1996) hypothesised that the likelihood of individuals becoming depressed was dependent on how much control they felt they had over events in their life, ie. whether they were helpless to prevent these events recurring and taking place in other areas of their life. Chiverton *et al* found that 22% of the women were clinically depressed; a significant finding when the incidence of depression in the general population is approximately 6%.

The researchers wanted to test the hypothesis that females who can comply with treatment methods and have a greater sense of mastery over their UI will maintain a higher QoL than those with a poor sense of mastery. The research found that a sense of mastery over UI and raised self-esteem correlated with a higher sense of QoL and lower levels of depression. Ashworth *et al* (1993) supported this, finding that young women who did not present for help saw their UI as their own fault.

Valerius (1997) used the Incontinence Impact Questionnaire (IIQ) and the Urogenital Distress Inventory (UDI) (Ubersax *et al*, 1995) in a prospective study to describe the relationship between UI, activities of living and distress. The IIQ and UDI are two health-related QoL tools specifically designed for UI (*Figure 4.1*). Valerius' (1997) use of these previously validated tools which were developed by a nursing and medical group (Ubersax *et al*, 1995) who have a professional interest in UI and are often quoted within the literature (Bech, 1993; Jackson, 1997), lends credibility to the single-author study. A sample of 35 women with UI, aged from 28–45 years old, was studied. Valerius (1997) found that 43% of the women perceived a moderate to high level of distress in sexual relations. This figure may be slightly lower than might be expected due to 97% of the sample being married and possibly more able to cope with UI within a long-term relationship.

The effect of UI in social-sexual relationships is again demonstrated by Ashworth and Hagan (1993) whose respondents spoke of being ashamed and fearing that, 'nobody wants to sit next to you'. Ashworth and Hagan's respondents also mentioned not enjoying sex as much due to the feeling of being dirty.

Type of urinary incontinence and its affect on quality of life

The previously mentioned Norton *et al* (1988) study examined the causal relationship between the independent variable of 'worst urinary symptom' and the dependent variable of age. Their findings included a significant relationship between age and the worst symptom. In women under 35 years old, frequency was the most prevalent symptom; in the 35–49 age group, stress incontinence was the most reported symptom; in those aged between 50 and 64 years mixed symptoms were reported, and in the over 65 age group, urge incontinence was the worst symptom.

Urge incontinence is associated with neurological effects and can result in complete and involuntary bladder emptying, while with stress incontinence, where urinary loss is exhibited upon physical exertion such as coughing or lifting, the activity is usually under the women's control and the amount of urinary loss is dependent on cessation of the activity. Norton *et al*'s (1988) study leaves some of the questions unanswered: is there a correlation between the type of urinary symptom and a delay in seeking treatment? If Norton *et al*'s findings are looked at alongside those of Chiverton *et al* (1996) and Grimby *et al* (1993), who observed that patients who reported urge incontinence suffered the greatest loss in their perceived QoL, then it may be that delay in seeking help is associated with depression and feelings of helplessness.

The Incontinence Impact Questionnaire (long form)

Has urine leakage and/or prolapse affected:

1. Ability to do household chores (cooking, house cleaning, laundry)?
2. Ability to do usual maintenance or repair work in home or yard?
3. Shopping activities?
4. Hobby and pastime activities?
5. Physical recreation such as walking, swimming or other exercise?
6. Entertainment activities (movies, concerts)?
7. Ability to travel by car or bus less than 30 minutes from home?
8. Ability to travel by car or bus more than 30 minutes from home?
9. Going to places if you are not sure about available rest rooms?
10. Going on vacation?
11. Church or temple attendance?
12. Volunteer activities?
13. Employment (work) outside your home?
14. Having friends visit you in your home?
15. Participating in social activities outside your home?
16. Relationships with friends?
17. Relationships with family?
18. Ability to have sexual relations?
19. Way you dress?
20. Emotional health?
21. Physical health?
22. Sleep?
23. Does fear of odour restrict your activity?
24. Does fear of embarrassment restrict your activities?

In addition, does your problem cause you to experience any of the following feelings:

25. Nervousness or anxiety?
26. Fear?
27. Frustration?
28. Anger?
29. Depression?
30. Embarrassment?

Urogenital Distress Inventory (long form)

Do you experience, and if so, how much are you bothered by:

1. Frequent urination?
2. A strong feeling of urgency to empty your bladder?
3. Urine leakage related to the feeling of urgency?
4. Urine leakage related to physical activity, coughing or sneezing?
5. General urine leakage not related to urgency or activity?
6. Small amounts of urine leakage (drops)?
7. Large amount of urine leakage?
8. Night time urination?
9. Bed wetting?
10. Difficulty emptying your bladder?
11. A feeling of incomplete bladder emptying?
12. Lower abdominal pressure?
13. Pain when urinating?
14. Pain or discomfort in the lower abdominal or genital area?
15. Heaviness or dullness in the pelvic area?
16. A feeling of bulging or protrusion in the vaginal area?
17. Bulging or protrusion you can see in the vaginal area?
18. Pelvic discomfort when standing or physically exerting yourself?
19. Having to push on the vaginal walls to have a bowel movement?

Figure 4.1: Quality of life tools specifically designed for urinary incontinence.
Source: Ubersax *et al* (1995)

In the quantitative study by Grimby *et al* (1993) the QoL of a randomly selected group of females, aged between 65 and 84 years and with diagnosed UI, was examined using a generic QoL questionnaire, the Nottingham Health Profile, originally used in patients with osteoarthritis (Bech, 1993). The Nottingham Health Profile incorporates 38 questions covering the topics shown in *Table 4.1*. As the tool is generic, rather than incontinence-specific, it was validated

Table 4.1: Topics covered by the Nottingham Health Profile
Sleep
Pain
Energy
Physical morbidity
Social isolation
Emotional reaction
Source: Bech (1993)

using a control group from the general population who were not incontinent and who otherwise had no significant variable differences (eg. age, build, specific illnesses) from the incontinent group.

Grimby *et al* (1993) found that the incontinent group experienced significant social isolation. Furthermore, when the incontinent group was analysed by type of incontinence, those with urge incontinence displayed greater feelings of isolation than those with stress or mixed incontinence symptoms. Significant emotional disturbances were found in those with urge and mixed incontinence but not for those with stress incontinence. There was also a correlation between urge incontinence and sleep disturbances. This study confirms what health professionals in the continence field have recognised in practice — that detrusor instability with urge incontinence is often devastating for the individual due to the unpredictability and severity of the incontinent episode.

Within society there is a belief that incontinence is a part of child-bearing. Ashworth and Hagan (1993) noted that incontinence was viewed as a regrettable result of motherhood and a fact of life. This finding may offer another perspective to the wealth of evidence, as cited above, that has found stress incontinence to have less effect on the individual's QoL than urge incontinence.

Fonda *et al* (1995), in a randomised control trial, studied the impact of non-surgical and non-pharmacological treatment on the QoL of all over 60-year-olds who were referred to a continence clinic in Melbourne, Australia. The interventions included pelvic floor muscle exercises and fluid advice (the measurement tool is shown in *Figure 4.2*). The control group who did not receive any interventions showed no significant changes in response to the questions in *Figure 4.2*. Those in the active treatment group showed significant improvements both in their symptoms and in their QoL. Fonda *et al* (1995) found no correlation between improvements and whether the women had detrusor instability or stress incontinence. However, over 10% of the final sample died before completion of the study indicating that a proportion of the patients may have had other diseases that were not specified by the author. It may be, therefore, that patient perception of their QoL was not specifically related to their UI.

For each of the statements the patient was asked to rate his/her response using the standard scale:

0 = not at all
1 = a little
2 = a lot
3 = very much

Statements:

Incontinence affects my family relations
There is more laundry associated with incontinence
I am depressed about being incontinent
The smell of incontinence bothers me
I am embarrassed about being incontinent

Figure 4.2: Quality of life statements. Source: Fonda *et al* (1995)

The impact of healthcare interventions on quality of life

Most of the available research examines the affect of UI on the individual's QoL. There is less data available to demonstrate the impact of healthcare interventions for UI on QoL. However, Moore and Sutherst (1990), in examining the impact of detrusor instability (DI) on the psychoneurosis state of 53 females, postulated that if there was a causal relationship between DI and neurosis then individuals would be difficult to treat with the drug oxybutynin as, regardless of the efficacy of the drug, the neurosis would be the dominant factor in the bladder problem.

The aim of the study was to determine whether there was any kind of relationship between those who responded well to drug therapy and those who responded poorly. The researchers demonstrated a relationship between good responders to oxybutynin and a psychoneurosis score in keeping with the general population and a relationship between poor responders and a psychoneurosis score reflective of psychoneurotic outpatients. This study, an earlier piece of work than most of the similar studies undertaken, begins the difficult task of measuring the outcomes of treatment on the individual's holistic well-being.

Conclusion

It is possible that the difficulty in creating a tool that measures QoL sensitively lies in the fact that people's lives are complicated. With disease this complication is heightened. The difficulty in any study which uses improvements in clinical symptoms to demonstrate efficacy of healthcare interventions is that UI has different meanings to both individual sufferers and health workers. Ashworth and Hagan (1993) note that some people feel they, 'just leak... (and are) not incontinent'. Researchers used different eligibility criteria to define UI, ranging from once a week (Gallagher, 1998) to a duration of incontinence greater than two months (Fonda *et al*, 1995). Only when clinicians have an understanding of how UI and various modalities affect patients' holistic well-being can the efficacy of care be evaluated.

The correlation between UI and diminished QoL has implications for healthcare professionals. The findings from these studies need to be incorporated into nursing practice in order to promote the holistic well-being of women and to challenge the widely held misconception that UI is a part of being female, a part of having children and a part of growing old. Therefore, the culture of the medical and nursing profession has to change through re-education.

Recommendations

- More qualitative work needs to be undertaken by nurses and doctors using randomly selected samples to establish how UI impacts on the QoL of the population who are not presenting for treatment.
- Greater emphasis of the affect of UI upon QoL needs to be incorporated into the education of nurses and doctors.
- There needs to be more multidisciplinary recognition of one incontinence-specific tool (not yet agreed upon by healthcare professionals) to measure QoL within the clinic setting.

Key points

❖ Urinary incontinence (UI) in females is recognised as having an adverse effect on quality of life (QoL).

❖ UI remains a taboo subject for sufferers both within their social environment and in relationships with healthcare professionals.

❖ There is evidence to show that urge incontinence has a more adverse effect on the sufferer's QoL than stress incontinence.

❖ A well validated tool for measuring the impact of UI upon the individual's QoL has yet to be agreed upon.

References

Ashworth P, Hagan MT (1993) The meaning of incontinence: a qualitative study of non-geriatric urinary incontinence sufferers. *J Adv Nurs* **18**: 1415–23

Bech P (1993) *Rating Scales for Psychopatholoy, Health Status and Quality of Life.* Springer-Verlag, Berlin

Chiverton PA, Wells RN, Brink CA, Mayer MD (1996) Psychological factors associated with urinary incontinence. *Clin Nurs Spec* **10**(5): 229–33

Fonda D, Woodward M, D'Astoli M, Wai Fong C (1995) Sustained improvement of subjective quality of life in older community-dwelling people after treatment of urinary incontinence. *Age Ageing* **24**: 283–6

Gallagher M (1998) Urogenital distress and the psychosocial impact of urinary incontinence on elderly women. *Rehab Nurs* **23**(4): 192–7

Grimby A, Milsom I, Molander U, Wiklund I, Ekelund P (1993) The influence of urinary incontinence on the quality of life of elderly women. *Age Ageing* **3**: 82–9

Jackson S (1997) The patient with overactive bladder symptoms and quality of life. *Urology* **50** (Supplement 6A): 18–22

Kelleher J, Cardozo LD, Toozs-Hobson PM (1995) Quality of life and urinary incontinence. *Curr Op Obstetr Gynaecol* **7**: 404–8

Moore K, Sutherst J (1990) Response to treatment of detrusor instability in relation to psychoneurotic status. *Br J Urol* **66**: 486–90

Norton PA, MacDonald LD, Sedgwick PM, Stanton SL (1988) Distress and delay associated with urinary incontinence, frequency and urgency in women. *Br Med J* **297**: 1187–9

Norton, C (1996) *Nursing for Continence.* 2nd edn. Beaconsfield, Buckinghamshire

Smith C (1998) Attitudes of health workers to incontinence. *J Comm Nurs* **12**(4): 8–14

Ubersax J, Wyman J, Shumaker S, McClish D, Fantl J (1995) Short forms to assess life quality and symptom distress for urinary incontinence in women: the incontinence impact questionnaire and the urogenital distress inventory. *Neurol Urodynam* **14**: 131–9

Valerius A (1997) The psychosocial impact of urinary incontinence on women aged 25 to 45 years. *Urol Nurs* **17**(3): 96–103

World Health Organization (1984) *Health Promotion: A WHO Discussion Document on the Concept and Principles.* WHO, Geneva

Bibliography

Bech P (1996) *The Bech, Hamilton and Zun Scales for Mood Disorders: Screening and Listening.* 2nd edn. Springer, Berlin

Black N, Griffiths J, Pope C (1996) Development of a symptom severity index and a symptom impact index for stress incontinence in women. *Neurol Urodynam* **15**: 630–40

French B (1997) British studies which measure patient outcome 1990–1994. *J Adv Nurs* **26**: 320–8

Nnishizawa O (1997) Discussion: assessment of symptoms in patients with an overactive bladder. *Urology* **50** (Supplement 6A): 23

Nolan C (1997) Continence clinic: positive outcomes difficulties encountered. *Br J Comm Health Nurs* **2**(7): 356–61

Norton C (1997) Discussion: quality of life in patients with overactive bladder. *Urology* **50** (Supplement 6A): 23–4

Parahoo K (1997) *Nursing Research. Principles, Process and Issues.* Macmillan, London

Roberts L (1998) Stress incontinence. *J Comm Nurs* **12**(12): 16–8

Sarantakos S (1993) *Social Research.* Macmillan, Australia

Section two
Catheterisation and catheter care:
Evidence-based practice

5

Urinary catheters: selection, maintenance and nursing care

Elisabeth Stewart

Catheterisation is often undertaken without sufficient assessment, and the high rates of bacteriuria (10–20%) occurring in catheterised patients seem to be accepted (Ward *et al*, 1997). This chapter reviews catheter selection, maintenance and nursing care, highlighting problem areas and suggesting measures that may be taken to reduce the risk factors. A problem-solving approach, based on research evidence relating to catheter care, is presented. Often there is a simple solution to a problem, but treatments based on traditions or myths appear to be the first choice in many situations. This chapter aims to provide nurses with the evidence base required to establish and maintain a urinary drainage system safely.

Bladder catheterisation has a long history, dating back to 30 BC. There are reports of catheters made from dried reeds, palm leaves, animal skins and cheese glue (Cule, 1980). In the 1920s, Foley designed the inflation balloon to retain the catheter in the bladder and to act as a haemostat. Foley catheters are still in use today (Roe, 1991). Urinary catheters are an essential component of medical care, with up to 12% of patients being catheterised during their stay in hospital (Mulhall *et al*, 1988).

The Public Health Laboratory Service has explored the area of hospital-acquired infection (HAI) and found that infections of the urinary tract account for about 40% of HAIs and are commonly associated with catheterisation. Between 10 and 20% of catheterised patients develop bacteriuria and 2–6% of all patients develop symptoms of urinary tract infection (UTI) (Ward *et al*, 1997).

The risk of acquiring bacteriuria is approximately 5% for each day of catheterisation. Other major risk factors are absence of systemic antibiotics, catheter care violations, advanced age and debilitation. Women are at greater risk than men (Ward *et al*, 1997).

Because catheter-associated UTI is often asymptomatic and resolves spontaneously on removal of the catheter, it is generally assumed to be insignificant. However, a proportion of patients remain at risk of UTI for up to 30 days after removal of the catheter. Between 1% and 4% of catheterised patients with UTI develop bacteraemia, of whom 13–30% die. The infected urinary tract is the most common source of Gram-negative septicaemia in hospitalised patients (Ward *et al*, 1997).

It cannot be stressed enough that people do still die from urinary sepsis. Wherever possible, alternative techniques should be considered for the management of patients with urinary retention or incontinence (Stickler and Zimakoff, 1994).

Catheter selection

A urethral catheter is a hollow tube inserted into the urinary bladder for the purpose of draining urine or instilling fluids as part of medical treatment. In 1930, Foley perfected a technique for manufacturing a one-piece catheter and balloon by dipping and coagulating latex on metal forms. There are now a variety of urinary catheters available for use in different situations, but the Foley catheter is still the most commonly used.

Catheter selection is extremely important. The catheter selected should promote a high rate of patient tolerance and a low rate of infection and rejection.

It is vital that the person inserting the catheter is aware of the range of products available and their different functions. Catheters are available for short-, medium- or long-term use and for a variety of indications (*Table 5.1*).

Table 5.1: Indications for catheterisation	
Postoperatively	Commonly used following surgical procedures
	To promote healing
	To measure urine output accurately
Acute illness	To monitor urine output
Urinary retention	Short-term management until the outflow obstruction has been treated
	Long-term if surgery or treatment fails or is not possible
	Postoperatively, patients should not be left longer than 6–8 hours without passing urine. Jolly (1997) advocates intermittent catheterisation for this group; however, this was only a small study
Urinary incontinence	Long-term catheterisation should be a last resort and only be considered after a full investigation and trial of other available management methods
Terminally ill	Catheterisation may be the only means by which the carer can cope with problems such as pain, frequency of micturition or maintenance of dignity. This can make the difference between hospitalisation and home care
Others	To determine residual urine volume
	To empty the bladder, eg. before abdominal, pelvic or rectal surgery and before investigations
	When teaching intermittent self-catheterisation either for incontinence or stricture
	For intravesical instillation of drugs
Duration of catheter usage:	
Short-term	Up to 3 weeks
Medium-term	Up to 6 weeks
Long-term	Up to 12 weeks

Catheter materials

Bacteria colonise the internal surface of the catheter, resulting in the formation of a biofilm, commonly known as an encrustation. Mulhall (1991) defines a biofilm as a collection of micro-organisms and their extracellular products bound to a solid surface. The biofilm becomes thicker and larger as the micro-organisms multiply and spread, and can obstruct the lumen of the catheter.

The catheter material can influence the rate at which biofilms develop (Merritt and Chang, 1991). When selecting a urinary catheter, therefore, it is imperative to consider which of the various materials available is the most appropriate.

Plastic

Plastic catheters are often used following urological surgery. They are more rigid and permit good drainage of clots and debris. However, patients find them stiff and inflexible, causing urethral pain (Norton, 1996), spasm and leakage. They are therefore suitable for short-term use only.

Latex

Latex is a purified form of rubber and the softest of the catheter materials. It has a smooth surface which is prone to crust formation owing to rapid disruption of the surface during use. Latex has been shown to cause urethral irritation and should therefore only be considered when catheterisation is likely to be short-term (Edwards, 1983).

Nurses need to be aware of the increasing incidence of latex allergy. Woodward (1997) highlights the problems of latex catheters, including toxicity leading to urethritis and stricture formation, and encrustation.

Teflon-coated latex

This material consists of polytetrafluoroethylene (PTFE; Teflon) permanently bonded to latex. PTFE is inert, providing a smooth outer surface that is less likely to be rejected, thus reducing trauma, irritation and encrustation (Seth, 1988). PTFE-coated latex catheters are suitable for short- or medium-term use (Pomfret, 1993).

Silicone elastomer

Silicone elastomer catheters are made of latex that has been dipped in silicone elastomer. They are thought to reduce the rate of formation of some encrustations. Unfortunately, there have been reports of the elastomer coating flaking off and damaging the urethra. These catheters are suitable for short- or medium-term use (Roberts *et al*, 1993).

Pure silicone

Silicone is a very soft, inert material which causes minimal urethral irritation. Catheters made of pure silicone are thin walled and so provide a larger lumen than coated catheters (Ryan-Wooley, 1987). However, silicone allows diffusion, which leads to deflation of the balloon over a period of time and can result in dislodgement of the catheter (Getliffe, 1993). These catheters are suitable for long-term use.

Hydrogel coated

This type of catheter is made of latex which has been bonded to hydrogel. The hydrogel coating also allows secretions from the urethral mucosa to be absorbed into the catheter. The catheter softens, making it more pliable and comfortable. Hydrogel is inert and is reported to be resistant to bacterial colonisation and encrustation. These catheters are suitable for long-term use (Talja *et al*, 1990; Roberts *et al*, 1993).

Catheter tips

A number of different catheter tips, designed for specific uses, are available (*Figure 5.1*). The standard tip is straight, rounded and has two drainage eyes.

Size of the catheter

The smallest size of catheter that will drain the contents of the bladder should be selected (Norton, 1996). Catheter sizes are designated by Charrière gauge (Ch) which is a measure of the diameter of the

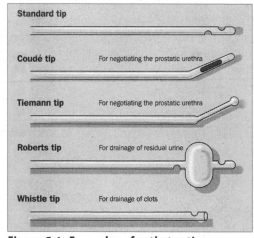

Figure 5.1: Examples of catheter tips

catheter in millimetres (1ch= 0.33mm diameter). Thus, a catheter of 12Ch has an outer diameter of 4mm.

A size 12–14Ch catheter is generally sufficient for both men and women.

Catheter sizes 16–18Ch should only be used if the patient has debris or mucus in the urine; and sizes in excess of 18Ch should be used only for patients with haematuria and clots which may occlude smaller lumens (Pomfret, 1996).

Larger catheters distend the elastic tissue of the urethral mucosa, so that it is unable to close its natural folds around the catheter. This leaves channels at either side which can lead to leakage of urine (Kennedy *et al*, 1983), pain due to bladder spasm (Roe and Brocklehurst, 1987) and blockage of urethral glands. All of these, in turn, can lead to infection, or ulceration of the bladder neck as a result of pressure.

The pressure exerted by a catheter that is too large can cause an increase in mucous secretions in the urethra. If these collect, they may become infected and lead to abscess and subsequent stricture formation. Pressure necrosis of the urethral meatus can also result from insertion of catheters that are too large (Edwards, 1983).

Balloon size

The 10ml balloon should be used routinely and inflated with 10ml of sterile water. Normal saline should not be used as salt particles can block the inflation channel and prevent balloon deflation. Likewise, tap water should not be used as it is not sterile and the density difference between tap water and urine means that osmosis can occur, leading to the transfer of bacteria (Bard, 1987). Inflating the balloon with air causes the balloon to float on the surface of the urine; the catheter tip then comes into contact with the bladder wall, causing irritation. Partial or over-inflation of the balloon is not recommended in routine catheterisation. It causes an asymmetrical balloon which can deflect the tip; this may then lie against the bladder wall, causing irritation and spasm (Belfield, 1988).

The 30ml balloon is designed specifically for use as a haemostat post-urological procedure, and should not be used for routine catheterisation. Large balloons can cause irritation of the urethral mucosa and trigone (the small triangular area between the two ureteric orifices and the internal urethral meatus) of the bladder. Contrary to popular belief (Crummey, 1989), this can give rise to spasm (Blannin and Hobden, 1980) and the bypassing of urine. With large balloons the drainage eye sits higher in the bladder, allowing a residual pool of urine to collect and therefore increasing the risk of infection (*Figure 5.2*).

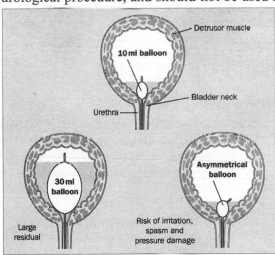

Figure 5.2: Normal and abnormal balloon placement

Catheter length

Both male (40cm) and female (23–25cm) length catheters are available. Female length catheters are much shorter and the reduced length outside the body results in less 'pulling' on the catheter. However, such catheters can be uncomfortable for obese women and produce pressure reactions around the groin.

Documentation

The insertion of an indwelling catheter carries many risks for the patient. Thorough documentation is therefore essential to ensure patient safety and correct monitoring. Each time a patient is catheterised, the following data must be recorded in the nursing notes:

- catheter type
- catheter size
- balloon size
- batch number
- expiry date
- date of insertion
- reason for catheterisation
- any difficulty on insertion
- volume of urine drained
- signature of person inserting the catheter.

Batch number and expiry date should be recorded so that in the event of a fault in a catheter, it can be reported to the manufacturer and/or Department of Health and be easily traced. Thorough documentation enables future carers to assess a patient's tolerance to his/her catheter and ensures continuity of care.

Drainage systems

The most common complications seen in catheterised patients are UTI and encrustation (Getliffe, 1994). When considering drainage systems, these risk areas need to be minimised as much as possible. Wilson and Coates (1996) showed that the use of a closed urinary drainage system reduced the incidence of UTI. A closed/link drainage system, which enables the bag to be emptied without unnecessary disconnection, is therefore recommended.

Whenever possible, patients should be allowed to choose a system that suits their needs. A closed system consists of a continuous catheter and collection device. This prevents disconnection from the catheter and plays a large part in reducing the rate of infection.

A link system consists of a leg bag (for use during the day) and a 2-litre non-drainable or drainable urine bag (for use during the night). The 2-litre urine bag is attached directly to the leg bag overnight and then removed in the morning. This system is more comfortable for the patient as it permits extra volume and extension to the system during the night. The closed system is still maintained. Where possible, a system that the patient can manage his/herself — even while in hospital — should be chosen.

The Department of Health (1992) recommends that urine drainage bags should be changed approximately every 5–7 days. Reid *et al* (1982) showed that there are no advantages to changing bags (attached directly to a catheter) more frequently.

Catheter valves

Catheter valves allow drainage of urine from a catheterised bladder without the need for a permanently attached drainage bag. The catheter valve must be released regularly to prevent over-distension of the bladder. Valves are therefore only suitable for patients who:

- have good manual dexterity
- can feel a full bladder
- are mentally aware
- are mobile
- have adequate bladder capacity.

Catheter valves are inappropriate for people with detrusor overactivity, ureteric reflux or renal impairment (Fader *et al*, 1997).

Catheter maintenance

Bladder washouts

Bladder washout comprises the instillation of a solution into the bladder via a catheter. The use of a bladder washout is a medical decision and the procedure must only be performed following, and according to, a medical prescription.

Prophylactic bladder washout is not generally recommended, owing to the risk of introducing further infection each time the closed system is disrupted. However, for repeated catheter blockages and encrustations, the use of bladder washouts should be considered (see *Chapter 10*).

A number of different solutions for bladder washout, with different actions (Getliffe, 1994) (*Table 5.2*), are available.

Table 5.2: Solutions used for bladder washouts	
Bladder washout	**Indications**
Sodium chloride 0.9%	Used when a purely mechanical effect is required for the removal of small bits of debris or small blood clots Can be used as required
Solution G (citric acid 3.23%)	Used to maintain patency of the catheter by dissolving encrustations and aiding re-acidification of urine. PH indicator papers can be used to assess the pH of urine and therefore the necessity for use of the solution (eg. pH>7.4) If patient's urine frequently returns to the alkaline state then solution R should be used (this reduces the number of times the closed system is broken) Can be used between twice daily and once weekly, depending on the severity of the encrustation
Solution R (citric acid 6%)	Used to unblock an encrusted catheter For use before removal of catheter to prevent trauma from encrustations To maintain patency of catheter by dissolving encrustations and aiding re-acidification of urine Can be used between twice daily and once weekly, depending on the severity of the encrustation
Chlorhexidine 0.02%	Aimed at reducing bacterial growth in the bladder Research has not found chlorhexidine bladder washouts to be beneficial. They do not eradicate established urinary tract infections and may lead to the development and selection of resistant organisms

Cranberry juice

Over the years, cranberry beverages have been thought to be useful in reducing bacterial infections of the bladder. Sobota (1984) showed that cranberry juice was effective in inhibiting bacterial adherence to mucosa and inhibiting the growth of yeast. Its mode of action and long-term effects are not known.

Unlike antibiotic therapy, it has no known side-effects at normal doses. It is a natural substance and is not licensed as a medicine. For patients who dislike the taste, it is also available in capsule form.

Cranberry juice is a natural and comparatively safe remedy, with the potential to provide symptomatic relief to many patients with UTI, urinary stones or excessive mucus formation (Busttil Leaver, 1996).

There is a risk of kidney stone formation if large amounts of cranberry juice are consumed. Individuals are therefore normally advised to drink only two glasses a day (approximately 400ml in total); at present there appear to be no side-effects from drinking this amount (Nazarko, 1995). Research relating to the role of cranberry juice in preventing bladder infection is limited; this is an area where further research would be beneficial.

Discharge from hospital with a catheter *in situ*

With the increasing number of patients being cared for in the community, it is vital that patients and carers are given comprehensive instructions on catheter care. Liaison with community health professionals is essential and will ensure that seamless care is provided. All patients who are to be discharged with a catheter *in situ* (whether permanent or temporary) require the following:

- district nurse referral: this should include documentation of the reasons for discharge with a catheter *in situ*, date of catheter insertion, when the catheter needs changing, type and size of catheter and balloon size
- discharge pack: this should contain at least one leg bag, five night bags and one pair of leg straps
- patient information leaflet
- knowledge of how to care for the catheter independently (or carer if appropriate)
- knowledge of how to recognise the onset of problems such as catheter blockage and infection
- contact telephone number for emergencies.

Troubleshooting

Bleeding: If there are only a few specks, it could be that the delicate lining of the urethra has been scratched during catheterisation and there is nothing to worry about. However, if the bleeding is persistent or becomes heavy, medical help should be sought.

Infection: Symptoms of infection include cloudy or foul-smelling urine, burning pain on passing urine and/or an elevated temperature, and rigors. If infection is suspected, send a urine sample for culture. Treat with antibiotics as indicated by the results and as prescribed by the doctor. Recommend a high intake of fluids, including cranberry juice.

No urine draining: Check that tubing is not kinked; check for constipation (pressure on the urethra can block the catheter and inflation channel); check that drainage system is below waist level; and check that tubing is not blocked (see below).

Urinary bypassing: Management of this problem is summarised in *Table 5.3*.

Table 5.3: Management of urinary bypassing in the catheterised patient	
Cause	**Management**
Encrustation and blocking	Bladder washout Replace catheter
Twisted tubing	Change position Unkink tubing
Constipation	Relieve constipation Dietary advice
Bladder spasm	Replace catheter with a smaller size catheter Consider anticholinergic or muscle relaxant medication
Bladder irritation	Increase fluid intake Commence antibiotics only if systemic symptoms present
Bladder calculi	Confirm by x-ray

Cramping pain: Usually settles after 24 hours. If pain persists it is usually due to an unstable bladder, with contractions causing discomfort (bladder spasms). Consider using anticholinergic drugs.

Urethral discomfort: This is caused by mechanical distension of the urethra resulting from too large a catheter or occlusion of the paraurethral glands leading to infection, urethritis and offensive discharge around the catheter. Consider changing to a smaller catheter.

Unable to deflate balloon: Check that patient is not constipated. Check non-return valve on the inflation channel; if it is jammed, use a needle and syringe to aspirate by means of the inflation arm above the valve. If this fails, refer to a urologist.

Do not attempt to cut the catheter or inflation channel or burst the balloon by overinflation.

Conclusion

Urinary catheterisation is not without complications and is associated with significant morbidity and, at times, mortality. The most problematic complication is bacteriuria. This chapter has highlighted evidence-based steps that should be taken when caring for a patient with an indwelling urinary catheter. If followed, the incidence of bacteriuria and other complications should be significantly reduced, benefiting both the patient and the hospital.

Key points

❖ Irrespective of gender, catheter size should be the smallest possible, usually 12 or 14Ch.

❖ Balloon size should never exceed 10ml (unless post-prostatic surgery).

❖ Short-term catheters must only stay *in situ* for a maximum of three weeks; long-term catheters for a maximum of three months.

❖ Maintain a closed drainage system at all times.

❖ Keep drainage bags below the level of the bladder.

❖ Overnight drainage bags should be attached to the outlet tap of a leg bag. Do not disconnect leg bags for overnight drainage.

❖ Remember that urinary tract infection remains the most common hospital-acquired infection.

References

Bard (1987) *Management and Care of Catheters and Collection Systems.* Bard, Crawley

Belfield (1988) Urinary catheter balloon volume. *Br Med J* **296**: 836 7

Blannin JP, Hobden J (1980) The catheter of choice. *Nurs Times* **76**: 2092–3

Busttil Leaver R (1996) Cranberry juice. *Profess Nurse* **11**(8). 525–6

Cule J (1980) Forerunners of Foley. *Nurs Mirror* **150**(5): 1–6

Crummey V (1989) Ignorance can hurt. *Nurs Times* **85**(21): 67–8

Edwards LE (1983) Post catheterisation urethral strictures. A clinical and experimental study. *Br J Urol* **55**: 53–6

Fader M, Pettersson L, Brooks R (1997) A multicentre comparative evaluation of catheter valves. *Br J Nurs* **6**(7): 359–67

Getliffe KA (1993) Care of urinary catheters. *Nurs Standard* **7**(44). 31–4

Getliffe KA (1994) The use of bladder wash-outs to reduce urinary catheter encrustation. *Br J Urol* **73**(6): 696–700

Jolly S (1997) Intermittent catheterisation for post-operative urine retention. *Nurs Times* **93**(33): 46–7

Kennedy A, Brocklehurst JC, Lyle MDW (1983) Factors related to the problems of long-term catheterisation. *J Adv Nurs* **8**: 202–12

Mulhall A (1991) Biofilms and urethral catheter infections. *Nurs Standard* **5**(18): 26–9

Mulhall AB, Chapman RG, Crow RA (1988) The acquisition of bacteriuria. *Nurs Times* **84**(4): 61–2

Nazarko L (1995) The therapeutic uses of cranberry juice. *Nurs Standard* **9**(34): 33–5

Norton C (1996) *Nursing for Continence.* Beaconsfield Publishers Ltd, Beaconsfield

Pomfret I (1993) Selecting catheters. *Community Outlook* April: 43–4

Pomfret I (1996) Catheters: design, selection and management. *Br J Nurs* **5**(4): 245–51

Reid RI, Pead PJ, Webster O, Maskell R (1982) Comparison of urine bag changing regimes in the elderly catheterised patients. *Lancet* **ii**: 754–6

Roberts JA, Kaack MB, Fussell EN (1993) Adherence to urethral catheters by bacteria causing nosocomial infections. *Urology* **41**(4). 338–42

Roe B (1991) Looking at the evidence. *Nurs Times* **87**(37): 72–4

Roe B, Brocklehurst JC (1987) Study of patients with indwelling catheters. *J Adv Nurs* **12**(6): 713–18

Ryan-Wooley B (1987) *Aids for the Management of Incontinence.* King's Fund, London

Seth C (1988) Catheters ring the changes. *Community Outlook* **May**: 12–14

Sobota AE (1984) Inhibition of bacterial adherence by cranberry juice: potential use for the treatment of urinary tract infections. *J Urol* **131**: 1013–16

Stickler DJ, Zimakoff J (1994) Complications of urinary tract infections associated with devices used for long term bladder management. *J Hosp Infect* **28**: 177–94

Talja M, Korpela A, Jarvi K (1990) Comparison of urethral reaction to full silicone, hydrogel-coated and siliconised latex catheters. *J Urol* **66**(6): 652–7

Ward V, Wilson J, Taylor L, Cookson B, Glynn A (1997) *Preventing Hospital-Acquired Infection: Clinical Guidelines.* Public Health Service Laboratory, HMSO, London

Wilson M, Coates D (1996) Infection control and urine drainage bag design. *Profess Nurse* **11**(4): 245–52

Woodward S (1997) Complications of allergies to latex urinary catheters. *Br J Nurs* **6**(14): 786–93

6

Catheterisation: a need for improved patient management

Linda Winson

The complications arising from catheterisation of the urinary bladder have been extensively researched and reviewed. It is widely accepted that, because of inherent risks, catheterisation is a last resort in the management of urinary incontinence. However, anecdotal evidence suggests that the incidence of long-term catheterisation for this purpose is increasing, particularly for the management of highly dependent patients in the community. Although catheterisation is a common procedure, a high level of nursing knowledge and skill is required to achieve effective and safe management. This chapter reviews the principles of catheter management and the nurse's responsibility to the catheterised patient.

Catheterisation is not a new procedure. It has been used for centuries in its simplest form for the intermittent relief of urinary retention. Primitive instruments made from reeds and various metals have been superseded by high-tech catheters designed to minimise the complications caused by the introduction of a foreign body into the urinary bladder. Catheterisation can be intermittent for episodic drainage of the bladder, or continuous.

Intermittent catheterisation is the technique of choice for individuals with neuropathic or hypotonic bladders associated with voiding difficulties and retention (Haynes, 1994). An advantage of intermittent catheterisation is that, for appropriate individuals, it can be performed independently; consequently, morale and confidence, which are frequently undermined by bladder dysfunction, improve in those who master the technique (Murray *et al*, 1984). The incidence of infection with intermittent catheterisation is reported to be lower than that associated with indwelling catheters (Hunt and Whitaker, 1984). Intermittent catheterisation requires separate consideration and is beyond the scope of this chapter.

Continuous catheter drainage

Catheters that are retained within the bladder are held in position by an inflated balloon and are known generically as Foley catheters after FB Foley who developed this system in the mid-1930s. Continuous catheter drainage is classified as: short-term 1–7 days; mid-term 7–28 days; and long-term 28 days or more (Slade and Gillespie, 1985). Catheters are also classified according to the use for which they are designed, and the quality of the materials from which they are made determine the classification. It is important that catheters of the most appropriate type, gauge, length and balloon size are selected for particular uses and patient needs (*Figure 6.1*).

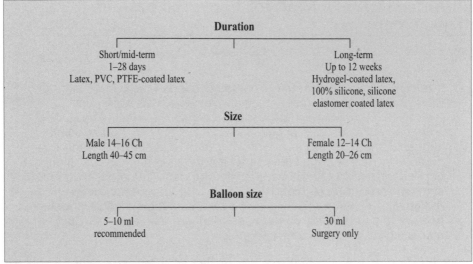

Figure 6.1: Catheter selection (PVC=polyvinyl chloride; PTFE=polytetrafluorethylene)

Catheters are inserted into the bladder via the natural channel of the urethra or through a suprapubic incision. Urethral catheterisation remains the most common technique, although the suprapubic route is becoming more popular; the advantages of the latter route include ease of re-catheterisation, no urethral trauma, less obstruction to sexual activity, greater patient comfort and urethral voiding can be retained where necessary (Iacovou, 1994). The introduction of an indwelling catheter by either route is a sterile procedure.

Catheter outlets are connected to a closed drainage system which facilitates continuous drainage, the collection of urine into a bag, and emptying of the bag without disconnection from the catheter. Patients, other than those with very restricted mobility, use a linked system. This comprises a sterile leg bag which is securely attached to the leg by straps, elasticated sleeve or holster during the day, and at night time is connected to a 2-litre drainage bag supported on a stand or hanger. For patients who are confined to bed or with very limited mobility, the closed system will consist of a sterile, drainable 2-litre bag attached directly to the catheter. As cross-infection is most likely to occur during bag changing and bag emptying (Platt *et al*, 1982), it is recommended that closed drainage systems remain intact for 5–7 days (Department of Health, 1992). Link night bags can be re-used if washed and drained dry for patients living in their own homes, as the risk of cross-infection is low (Getliffe, 1993).

There is a wide range of drainage bags available and bags should be selected to accommodate patient dexterity, output volume, comfort and preference. Essential features should include a non-return flap valve, conveniently operated outlet tap at the bottom of the bag and a sample port for specimen collection (Falkiner, 1993).

The use of catheter valves has recently become more popular (Roe, 1990a). A catheter valve is a small device that connects directly to the catheter outlet and is similar to a leg bag tap. For suitably aware and dextrous patients with a good bladder capacity, a catheter valve can be the means of dispensing with drainage systems, as urine is stored in the bladder and drained intermittently by releasing the valve. Several makes of catheter valves are available in the UK, three of which are on Drug Tariff; Bard Flip-Flo catheter valve, Seton Scholl catheter valve, Sims Portex Uro-Flo catheter valve. Most valves allow connection to drainage bags if required (Fader *et al*, 1997). The advantages and disadvantages of this system have not yet been fully researched, but will be of interest, particularly when related to incidence of infection (*Table 6.1*).

Table 6.1: Catheter valves: potential advantages and disadvantages	
Advantages	More discreet
	More comfortable
	Less traction exerted on bladder neck and urethra
	May help to retain bladder tone as the bladder fills and empties intermittently
	Allow more independence
	Most valves can be attached to drainage bags if necessary
	Can be used with urethral or suprapubic catheters
Disadvantages	Risk of overdistension of the bladder
	Unsuitable for people with low bladder capacity, hyperreflexia, ureteric reflux or renal impairment
	Users must have sufficient manual dexterity to open and close the catheter valve
	Users must have good cognitive ability to ensure that catheter valves are released regularly
	Users must have sufficient mobility to access the appropriate place and/or equipment to facilitate regular bladder emptying
	No current research into risk of infection

The catheter valves available on Drug Tariff are licensed by the Department of Health for five to seven days use and this corresponds with the recommendations of most manufacturers.

Incidence of catheterisation

Catheterisation is a common procedure and catheterised patients are widely distributed across all areas of care. The prevalence has been established as 10%

of patients in hospital (Mulhall *et al*, 1988), and 4% of patients receiving nursing services at home (Getliffe and Mulhall, 1991).

The majority of patients catheterised in the acute hospital setting have a short-term or mid-term urethral catheter inserted, while those in the community are more likely to have long-term catheters inserted.

Indications for catheterisation are to facilitate drainage, investigation and treatment (*Table 6.2*).

Table 6.2: Indications for catheterisation		
Indwelling	Retention	Acute
		Chronic
	Incontinence	Intractable problem resistant to treatment
		Patient unfit for treatment
	To maintain bladder drainage following surgery, eg. prostatectomy, cystoplasty	
	Monitoring urine output	
Intermittent	Treatment, eg. intravesical chemotherapy, prolonged bladder distension	
	Investigations, eg. cystometry, micturating cystourethrography	
Source: Iacovou (1993)		

Research and professional opinion support the view that catheterisation should be a last resort in the management of incontinence and that the condition should be established as intractable before such measures are considered (Falkiner, 1993). As other techniques and appliances have become available, catheterisation is now used less than previously, for the management of incontinence (Roe, 1993). However, methods such as penile sheaths, male collection appliances and absorbent body-worn products often require levels of physical dexterity, mental agility or adequate assistance from a responsible carer that are not always available.

An ageing population and the emphasis on care in the community for individuals with chronic disease could make the use of long-term catheterisation in the management of incontinence more likely.

Although the decision to catheterise should be based on clinical need, the potential for this decision to be influenced by increasing pressures on resources and costs in hospital and community is considerable.

Complications of catheterisation

Infection

Urinary infection is the most common complication of catheterisation. Significant microbial counts can be detected in most patients three days after catheterisation (Bach *et al*, 1990). The risk of developing bacteriuria is estimated by Garibaldi *et al* (1974) as 8.1% for each day that the catheter remains in place and bacteriuria is virtually inevitable within three to four weeks (Jewes *et al*, 1988).

Bacteria may be introduced into the bladder during catheterisation by migration of organisms along the peri-urethral space, or via the catheter lumen, from contaminated drainage bags or catheter outlet connections (Mulhall *et al*, 1993).

Scrupulous attention to handwashing and use of disposable gloves by carers when handling catheters or emptying catheter bags may prevent infection from exogenous organisms (eg. *Serratia spp.* and *Pseudomonas aeruginosa*) found in the environment and on hands. Infection by endogenous faecal or urethral micro-organisms (eg. Gram-positive cocci and *Klebsiella*) is more difficult to prevent (Garibaldi *et al*, 1980). Meatal cleansing with various antiseptic and antibacterial solutions has been advocated to try to prevent entry of bacteria at the meatal junction. However, procedures have proved ineffective (Desautels, 1960; Burke *et al*, 1983) and it is recommended that simple meatal cleansing with soap and water to prevent encrustation is sufficient (Falkiner, 1993).

Management of the short-term catheter should focus on the prevention of infection through adherence to strict standards of hygiene, the maintenance of closed drainage systems and early removal of the catheter where possible. As antibiotic therapy is likely to be ineffective for bacteriuria, it should be reserved for the treatment of systemic or symptomatic infection (Gillespie, 1986). Falkiner (1993), however, found a significant reduction in the incidence of septicaemia following any manipulation (including catheter removal) of the catheterised urinary tract if urine was cultured to isolate and appropriately treat infection before performing the procedure.

Infection is an inevitable consequence of long-term catheterisation. Micro-organisms colonise the surfaces of catheters and drainage bags, forming a biofilm; this is defined by Mulhall (1991) as 'a collection of micro-organisms and their extracellular products bound to a solid surface' which thickens as the micro-organisms multiply. As the living micro-organisms are located deep within the matrix of the biofilm they are generally unaffected by treatment with antibiotics. Infections are mostly asymptomatic as a protective layer of mucus on the bladder wall limits bacterial invasion and helps to prevent systemic infection (Getliffe, 1993). Systemic and local antibiotic therapy should only be administered if the patient develops symptoms of infection, such as pyrexia, haematuria, nausea, vomiting, malaise and confusion as inappropriate use may lead to the development of and exposure to more pathogenic organisms (Norton, 1986).

Bypassing

Leakage of urine from around a catheter can be caused by kinked tubing, restrictive clothing, constipation or bladder spasm. Drainage can be impaired by over-full or incorrectly positioned catheter bags, which may also result in bypassing. Simple mechanical obstruction should always be considered in the first instance. Patients with long-term catheters inserted can be divided into two groups; blockers and non-blockers (Kunin *et al*, 1987). Blockers quickly develop dense catheter encrustation, invariably in the presence of a high urinary pH. If the pH remains low, there is significantly less risk of a patient becoming a blocker (Hedelin *et al*, 1991). Infection by urease-producing organisms, eg. *Proteus mirabilis*, may lead to urinary alkalisation and precipitation of mineral salts (struvite) on the catheter and its lumen (Getliffe, 1994).

However, Hedelin *et al* (1991) found that the presence of urease producers was not associated with a high pH or greater precipitation in all patients, and concluded that encrustation appears also to depend on individual factors, such as urinary composition, and not just the presence of urease-producing micro-organisms. Attempts to lower urine osmolality and maintain a high diuresis by a high fluid intake are considered to have little beneficial effect. Similarly, the ingestion of acidifying agents, eg. cranberry juice or ascorbic acid, is of little benefit in preventing catheter encrustation (Getliffe, 1993). However, Roe (1993) suggests that increased diuresis will help to flush micro-organisms out of the bladder. From her study of the effectiveness of bladder washouts in reducing catheter encrustation, Getliffe (1994) concludes that citric acid solutions (Suby G and Solution R) or mandelic acid may be beneficial in the management of recurrent catheter encrustation and blockage. This should be balanced against the known benefits of maintaining a closed drainage system.

Kunin *et al* (1987) suggest that catheter renewal should be individually planned, following systematic evaluation of the formation of encrustation, to prevent blockage and bypassing occurring.

Discomfort

A catheter is a foreign body and can cause discomfort. Many people experience catheter cramp when they are first catheterised. This results from irritation of the urethra and bladder and usually subsides within 24 hours, although it can persist in some people (Norton, 1986). Appropriate selection of catheter type and size will help to reduce the likelihood of this reaction (Roe and Brocklehurst, 1987). Prolonged urethral irritation can cause urethritis and possibly the eventual development of urethral strictures (Edwards *et al*, 1983).

Detrusor instability is frequently exacerbated or caused by the presence of a catheter in the bladder. This results in uninhibited bladder spasm, discomfort and the eventual bypassing of urine around the catheter. Anticholinergic medication may help to inhibit such unstable bladder contractions (Norton, 1986). Smaller gauge catheters and smoother biocompatible catheter surfaces, eg. silicone, teflon and hydrogel, are less likely to irritate the urethra and bladder wall

(Falkiner, 1993). Balloon size is also relevant to levels of bladder irritation and for long-term catheterisation should be 5–15ml capacity (Kunin, 1987).

Bladder spasm may cause particular problems in urethrally catheterised females with neurogenic bladder dysfunction. When females sit, pressure and friction are transmitted onto the urethral orifice. This tends to trap the catheter, which then exerts continuous traction on the bladder neck and urethra. This may result in bladder spasm that is sufficiently strong to cause expulsion of the catheter with the balloon inflated. Repeated episodes of catheter expulsion with the balloon inflated can lead to complete erosion of the bladder neck and urethra in females, and occasionally in males (Iacovou, 1994).

Interference with sexual function

The presence of a urethral catheter does not necessarily preclude sexual intercourse. Males are advised to tape the catheter back onto the shaft of the penis and/or hold it in place by covering it with a condom. Females are advised to tape the catheter up onto the abdomen (Winder, 1994). However, this may be associated with significant physical and psychological problems, such as trauma, infection, retrograde ejaculation (males), dyspareunia, impaired self-image, embarrassment, depression and loss of libido. It is advisable for a sexually active person or his/her partner to be instructed in the removal and replacement of the urethral catheter to facilitate unfettered intercourse; alternatively, suprapubic catheterisation may be preferred (Norton, 1986).

Although sexual function may be facilitated by appropriate catheter management, catheterisation will have an effect on the sexuality of all individuals experiencing it. Anders (1993) states that sexuality is mainly about the actual person, his/her personality and self-concept. Holistic patient assessment must include sexuality; however, Jacobson (1974) found that nurses are reluctant to address it.

Responsibilities of the nurse

Although the decision to initiate catheter drainage should be made by the medical practitioner responsible for the patient's care (Norton, 1986), this is frequently influenced by nursing assessment, particularly in the management of patients with chronic medical conditions. In addition, medical practitioners frequently depend on nursing advice for the selection of appropriate catheters and drainage systems.

Over 50% of catheters are inserted by medical staff (Mulhall *et al*, 1993). This undoubtedly reflects the higher incidence of catheterisation in acute hospitals than in the community, where the majority of catheterisations are carried out by nurses. It is, therefore, the nurse's responsibility to carry out a holistic assessment, which requires knowledge of the biological, physiological and social implications associated with catheterisation (Clarke, 1995), and to develop the clinical skills that will enable him/her to catheterise patients safely and plan proactive, ongoing care. Although trained nurses have responsibility for catheterisation and catheter management, day-to-day care is likely to be provided by untrained personnel (formal or informal) or the patients themselves. The primary nurse should ensure that carers have sufficient knowledge, ability and support to manage the catheter system effectively and with confidence.

Management of the catheterised patient

The aims of catheter management are listed in *Table 6.3*.

Table 6.3: The aims of catheter management
To prevent or minimise the complications related to catheterisation
To promote the independence, comfort and dignity of the patient
To ensure that the patients and carers understand, and can cope safely with, the catheter and drainage systems through: holistic assessment of the patient's needs; patient education and shared decision-making; selection of the correct type and size of catheter; aseptic catheterisation technique; maintenance of a closed drainage system; effective handwashing before and after handling catheter or drainage bags; meatal hygiene; bladder washout regimen, if indicated; and planned re-catheterisation programme

Patient education

The importance of the role of nurses as educators has been identified by Roe (1992) and Norton (1986), particularly in the promotion of continence and management of incontinence.

Nurses have an unequalled opportunity to inform and educate patients and carers. However, Roe and Brocklehurst (1987) claim that the education of patients and carers about catheter management has been a neglected aspect of practice, with little information and explanation being given to them. Roe (1990b) found that patients who received an education programme and information booklet had significantly better knowledge of catheter management and how to minimise the associated risks. It was concluded that patients benefited from early instruction and subsequent reinforcement of information.

Nurse education

Mulhall *et al* (1993) describe nursing as a traditional discipline based on historical experience rather than research-based evidence and nurses as having more diverse levels of skill, knowledge and education than possibly any other profession. It has also been suggested that it is not possible for all nurses to carry out patient education as they do not have sufficient knowledge or the teaching skills required (Luker and Caress, 1989). Post-basic nurse education should provide the opportunity for all qualified nurses to enhance their knowledge and skills through training in specialised areas of practice and that standards of practice should be based on scientific evidence (Clarke, 1995).

Conclusion

Catheterisation in acute care will always be indicated for clinical management purposes. The instigation of long-term catheterisation should be based on an informed holistic assessment, taking into account the potential associated risks and complications. Nurse education should equip them with the knowledge and skills to plan proactive catheter management and with the ability to teach and inform patients. Local policy and procedure should be developed and be based on scientific evidence.

Many booklets are available from manufacturers of catheters and drainage systems, for nurses and patients and carers. Most are written by, or in association with, experts in clinical practice and provide research-based information on all types of catheterisation and aspects of catheter management. Every catheterised patient should be provided with written information on catheter care and, in case of need, be supplied with a contact name and phone number. Examples are: *Catheter Care. A Guide for Users and their Carers*. SIMS Portex Ltd, Hythe, Kent, CT21 6JL. Tel: 01303 260551; *A Guide for Nurses. Management and Care of Catheters and Collection Systems*. Bard Ltd, Forest House, Brighton Rd, Crawley, West Sussex, RH11 9BP. Tel: 01293 529555; *You and Your Catheter*. Simpla Plastics Ltd, Tubiton House, Oldham, OL1 3HS. Tel: 0800 526177.

Key points

❖ Catheterisation of the urinary bladder is frequently performed in hospitals and in the community.

❖ The most common indications for catheterisation are bladder outlet obstruction and incontinence.

❖ The demand on limited resources and the emphasis on care in the community provide the potential for an increase in the use of catheters for the management of intractable incontinence.

❖ Catheterisation is an invasive procedure and carries an increased risk of morbidity and mortality.

❖ There is an urgent need to provide information and training to all who are involved in catheter care.

References

Anders K (1993) Open communication can restore self-esteem: sexuality issues related to cystectomy for stoma formation. *Prof Nurse* **8**(10): 638–43

Bach D, Hesse A, Prauge CH (1990) Prophylaxis against encrustation and urinary tract infection with indwelling transurethral catheters. *Urol/Nephrol* **2**(1): 25–32

Burke JP, Jacobson JA, Garibaldi RA, Conti MT, Alling DW (1983) Evaluation of meatal care with polyantibiotic ointment in prevention of urinary catheter-associated bacteriuria. *J Urol* **120**: 331–4

Clarke M (1995) Nursing and the biological sciences. *J Adv Nurs* **22**: 405–6

Department of Health (1992) *Drug Tariff*. HMSO, London

Desautels RE (1960) Aseptic management of catheter drainage. *N Engl J Med* **263**: 189–91

Edwards LE, Lock R, Powell C, Jones P (1983) Post catheterisation urethral structures: a clinical and experimental study. *Br J Urol* **55**: 53–6

Fader M, Pettersson L, Brooks R, Dean G, Wells M, Cottenden A, Malone-Lee J (1997) A multicentre comparative evaluation of catheter valves. *Br J Nurs* **6**(7): 359–67

Falkiner FR (1993) The insertion and management of indwelling urethral catheters — minimising the risk of infection. *J Hosp Infect* **25**: 79–90

Garibaldi RA, Burke JP, Dickman ML, Smith CB (1974) Factors predisposing to bacteriuria during indwelling urethral catheterisation. *J Med* **291**: 216–9

Garibaldi RA, Burke JP, Britt MR, Miller WA, Smith CB (1980) Meatal colonisation and catheter-associated bacteriuria. *N Engl J Med* **303**: 316–18

Getliffe KA (1993) Informed choices for long-term benefits: the management of catheters in continence care. *Prof Nurse* **9**(2): 122–6

Getliffe KA (1994) The use of bladder wash-outs to reduce urinary catheter encrustation. *Br J Urol* **73**: 696–700

Getliffe KA, Mulhall AB (1991) The encrustation of indwelling catheters. *Br J Urol* **67**: 337–41

Gillespie WA (1986) Antibiotics in catheterised patients. *J Antimicrob Chemother* **18**: 149–51

Haynes S (1994) Intermittent self-catheterisation — the key facts. *Prof Nurse* **10**(2): 100–4

Hedelin H, Brah CG, Eckerdal G, Lincoln K (1991) Relationship between urease-producing bacteria, urinary pH and encrustation on indwelling urinary catheters. *Br J Urol* **67**: 527–31

Hunt GM, Whitaker RH (1984) Intermittent self-catheterisation in adults. *Br Med J* **289**: 467–8

Iacovou JW (1993) Urethral catheterisation of the urinary bladder. *Hosp Update* **19**(8): 457–9

Iacovou JW (1994) Suprapubic catheterisation of the urinary bladder. *Hosp Update* **20**(3): 159–62

Jacobson I (1974) Illness and human sexuality. *Nurs Outlook* **22**(1): 50–3

Jewes LA, Gillespie WA, Leadbetter A (1988) Bacteriuria and bacteraemia in patients with long-term indwelling catheters — a domiciliary study. *J Med Microbiol* **26**: 61–5

Kunin CM (1987) *Detection, Prevention and Management of Urinary Tract Infections*. 4th edn. Lea and Febier, Philadelphia

Kunin CM, Chin QF, Chambers S (1987) Indwelling catheters in the elderly. Relation of catheter life to formation of encrustations in patients with and without blocked catheters. *Am J Med* **82**: 405–11

Luker A, Caress A (1989) Rethinking patient education. *J Adv Nurs* **14**(9): 711–18

Mulhall AB (1991) Biofilms and urethral catheter infections. *Nurs Standard* **5**(18): 26–8

Mulhall AB, Chapman RG, Crow RA (1988) The acquisition of bacteriuria. *Nurs Times* **84**(4): 61–2

Mulhall AB, King S, Lee K, Wiggington L (1993) Maintenance of closed urinary drainage systems: are practitioners more aware of the dangers? *J Clin Nurs* **2**: 135–40

Murray K, Lewis P, Blannis J, Sheppard A (1984) Clear intermittent self-catheterisation in the management of adult lower urinary tract dysfunction. *B J Urol* **56**: 379–80

Norton C (1986) *Nursing for Continence*. Beaconsfield Publishers, Beaconsfield

Platt R, Polk BF, Murdock B, Rosner B (1982) Mortality associated with nosocomial urinary tract infection. *New Engl J Med* **307**: 637–42

Roe (1990a) Do we need to clamp catheters? *Nurs Times* **86**(43): 66–7

Roe BH (1990b) Study of the effects of education on patients' knowledge and acceptance of their indwelling urethral catheters. *J Adv Nurs* **15**: 223–31

Roe BH (1992) Teaching patients and carers about continence. In: Roe BH, eds. *Clinical Nursing Practice: The Promotion and Management of Continence*. Prentice Hall, London: 177–95

Roe BH (1993) Catheter-associated urinary tract infection: a review. *J Clin Nurs* **2**: 197–203

Roe BH, Brocklehurst JC (1987) Study of patients with indwelling catheters. *J Adv Nurs* **12**: 713–8

Slade N, Gillespie WA (1985) *The Urinary Tract and the Catheter*. Wiley, New York

Winder A (1994) Incontinence and sexuality. *Community Outlook* **4**(8): 21–2

7

Indications for and principles of intermittent self-catheterisation

Willie Doherty

Intermittent self-catheterisation (ISC) or carer/nurse assisted intermittent catheterisation has developed over the past few years as a means of treating patients with bladder emptying problems. Initially the process was designed for patients with the dexterity to carry out the procedure; today, however, more nurses are trained in the technique and are therefore able to support people with coordination problems in carrying out the procedure. Education programmes on catheterisation are becoming increasingly popular and many district nurses have become skilled in its practice. This chapter describes some of the conditions that may be associated with bladder dysfunction and which warrant ISC. The support required from nurses in the planning, implementing, intervention and evaluation of a package of care are discussed. Simple advice such as avoiding constipation, monitoring urine to identify infection and general measures to improve hygiene all play a role in maintaining good health.

Intermittent self-catheterisation (ISC) is the act of passing a catheter into a poorly functioning bladder via the urethra in order to drain urine; the catheter is removed immediately afterwards. The technique is a way of reducing bladder symptoms resulting from accumulating urine which cannot be eliminated naturally. Incomplete bladder emptying can lead to bladder infection; in addition, high intravesicle pressure can cause damage to the upper urinary tract as a result of reflux to the kidneys (Winder, 1992).

ISC will benefit people with symptoms of difficulty voiding as well as those who have urinary frequency and urgency because their bladders are constantly nearly full (Herr, 1975; Perkash, 1975; Dionko *et al*, 1985). As there are no effective medications for improving bladder emptying ISC is deemed the best way of managing the problem (Fowler, 1998).

The procedure has been widely advocated for 20 years (Lapides *et al*, 1972, 1976) but actually dates back to 30 BC when Celsus acknowledged the importance of the procedure in *Disquisation De Medicina:*

> *Sometimes we are compelled to draw off urine by hand when it is not passed naturally. For this purpose bronze tubes are made.*

Avicenna, a urologist (AD 980–1037), recommended that catheters should be made from marine animal skins (Winder, 1992). Today, polyvinyl chloride (PVC) is more commonly used for single- and multiple-use catheters.

ISC can be carried out by all age groups (Winder, 1992) as either a 'one-off' procedure to measure a residual volume or a more long-term procedure to ensure bladder emptying.

If patients are unable to carry out the procedure for themselves the technique can be taught to carers. If a carer is to assume responsibility for the procedure, the nurse must be aware of his/her trust's local protocols in relation to consent before commencing any education package directed at carers. Education of carers must take place regularly and the patient's named nurse is responsible for ensuring that this takes place. Whenever healthcare professionals relinquish any aspect of care to non-professionals they must remember that they are still responsible for ensuring that the care is carried out effectively and safely.

Indications for intermittent self-catheterisation

The following are conditions and interventions that may necessitate the need for ISC:

Conditions

Underactive detrusor function (atonic or non-contractile bladder): With this condition the bladder fails to empty because normal voiding processes are interrupted between bladder and micturition centres in the brain. This causes urine to collect which may lead to the bladder becoming atonic. There is an added risk of urinary tract infection because of the accumulation of stale urine. The condition is most common in patients with neurological problems such as multiple sclerosis and in spinal injuries (Guttmann and Frankel, 1966).

Overactive urethral closure mechanism (detrusor sphincted dyssynergia): In normal voiding the bladder contracts and the sphincter relaxes. With detrusor sphincted dyssynergia the bladder and sphincter contract simultaneously. It can occur in people with neurological conditions such as multiple sclerosis (Murray *et al*, 1984).

Urethral obstruction (prostatic enlargement or urethral stricture): Prostatic obstruction causes the urethra to become narrowed which makes patients tighten their lower abdominal muscles to put pressure on the underlying bladder in order to empty it. This cannot be sustained and therefore bladder emptying becomes difficult resulting in poor flow, frequency and post-micturition dribble. Similar problems occur with urethral strictures caused by infection, trauma or a congenital abnormality: the urethra is narrowed and patients have to rely on abdominal pressure in order to void (Brocklehurst *et al*, 1968; Brocklehurst, 1977).

Neurological disorders (eg. multiple sclerosis): The bladder problems associated with neurological disorders such as multiple sclerosis are overactivity and incomplete emptying. Overactivity can be treated with anticholinergic medication (except in cases where incomplete emptying is also present). There are no effective medications for dealing with incomplete bladder emptying and therefore ISC is the best way of managing this problem (Fowler, 1998).

Diabetes mellitus (ie. incomplete emptying as a result of neuropathy): With diabetic patients there may be some neurological deficit caused by the progression of the disease. This may result in bladder emptying problems due to reduced bladder filling awareness. Where residual urine is present (see below) ISC may be indicated; this should be regulated and reduced as the volume of residual urine decreases (Herr, 1975; Perkash, 1975; Dionko *et al*, 1985).

Cerebrovascular accident: A cerebrovascular accident often results in poor bladder function. If there is residual urine volume (see below) a treatment plan needs to be devised in order to reduce this:

- residual urine is measured by passing a catheter and draining the bladder
- when (and if) the residual urine left in the bladder after voiding falls below 100–200ml, frequency of catheterisation is reduced
- it may only be necessary to catheterise once a day or once a week.

If residual urine remains higher than 120ml then ISC may be required long-term (Herr, 1975).

Spina bifida: Many patients with spina bifida have considerable bladder problems because of the disruption or incomplete connection between the micturition centre in the brain, and the spinal cord and bladder. This may lead to incontinence. ISC can be of considerable benefit to those with little or no bladder control as a means of developing continence and thus preventing the embarrassment of having to wear incontinence pads (Lapides *et al*, 1972).

Interventions

Surgical intervention (eg. colposuspension): A colposuspension can reduce the incidence of incontinence but there may be a greater chance of outflow obstruction (Getliffe and Dolman, 1997) which may indicate the need for ISC. This may only be necessary for a few weeks or months but in some cases the procedure may have to be carried out for life (Hilton, 1987).

Continent urinary diversions (eg. a Mitrofanoff): The Mitrofanoff urinary diversion may be performed when all other measures to correct incontinence, such as urethral catheterisation (indwelling and intermittent), have failed or there is congenital abnormality or trauma affecting the urethra or sphincter mechanism.

A Mitrofanoff is a catheterisable channel for the bladder. A stoma-type opening that is connected to the bladder, made from tissue such as the appendix, fallopian tube or a vein, is fashioned on the surface of the abdomen. The appendix can be inverted to act as a valve, thus preventing leakage. The position of the stoma is above the bladder level which also acts to prevent leakage. Some patients like to wear a stoma cap type device for security. The principle is to allow the bladder to act as a reservoir for urine so that the patient can catheterise the stoma in order to empty the bladder at regular intervals. The potential benefit of using the Mitrofanoff is that catheterisation is simplified, especially in the female patient. Recent modification has allowed the stoma to be hidden within the umbilicus giving excellent cosmetic results (Sumfest *et al*, 1993; Horowitz *et al*, 1995).

Assessment

In order to determine whether a patient is suitable for ISC some urologists advocate urodynamic studies, eg. the measurement of post-micturition residual volume (the volume that is left behind after the patient has passed urine) (Chapple and Christmas, 1990). This measurement can be made by either using ultrasound or passing a catheter into the bladder. Finding more than 100ml of urine indicates that the bladder is not emptying properly. It must be noted that urodynamic studies are not appropriate for all patients due to the invasive nature of the procedure (Fowler, 1998).

Before assessing whether patients are able to carry out ISC all nurses must ensure that they are competent to teach this skill. For example, they must have attended an appropriate education session and be familiar with local guidelines and protocols. Coloplast has developed a teaching-to-teach intermittent self-catheterisation package (Winder *et al*, 1997). This was produced to support a course on this subject which has gained RCN accreditation. (Further details can be obtained by contacting Coloplast: 01733 392061.)

Patients' suitability to carry out ISC as an ongoing care initiative is dependent on the following:

- manual dexterity
- ability to learn the task effectively
- motivation to continue with a procedure that will continue for a considerable period of time, even for the rest of the patients' lives
- awareness of the problems associated with ISC
- understanding of how to avoid associated problems, such as urinary tract infections.

The assessment process needs to develop at a pace dictated by the patient to ensure full understanding of the procedure. Permission must be sought from the GP or consultant before approaching the patient. Some patients may have heard about ISC from fellow sufferers and assumed that it is appropriate for their condition; however, this is not always the case.

Assessment involves the collection of data and information specifically related to each individual's problem of incontinence. Initially, a frequency volume chart is necessary to identify the number of times a person is voiding, the amount voided and the frequency of getting up at night to pass urine. Men with prostate problems have to go to the toilet often in the night but will only pass small amounts of urine. Flow rate measurement is very useful to identify an outflow obstruction and can be done quite easily in the clinical situation.

If the patient cannot come to the clinic, this can be done at home because the equipment is portable. Most continence advisers have access to a bladder scanner which is useful to record a residual urine or a maximum bladder capacity.

Assessment is time-consuming and some information may remain unobtainable on the initial assessment, mainly because patients are reticent about discussing their bladder problems. Assessment must therefore be regarded as an ongoing and cumulative process. Lengthy discussions with the patient may be necessary to identify any potential problems. For example:

- non-compliance with the procedure once it has been initiated
- poor dexterity resulting in failure of the patient to carry out the procedure
- reluctance of a related carer to be involved where the patient cannot catheterise
- taking shortcuts with hygiene, thus increasing the risk of urinary tract infection.

Nurses also need to assure themselves that the procedure is an appropriate form of treatment for the individual.

Educating patients

Patients must be given a basic knowledge of their anatomy and physiology so that they are reassured that this method of bladder emptying is safe and will not cause them any harm, providing they adhere to the care programme advised (*Figure 7.1*).

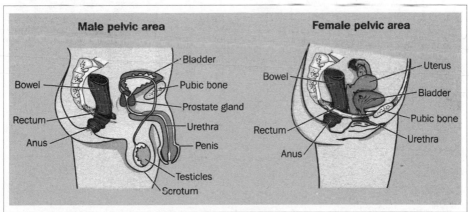

Figure 7.1: Anatomy of the male and female pelvic area. Understanding basic anatomy and physiology will help patients adhere to the care programme as they will be reassured that the procedure is safe

The concept of ISC is difficult to grasp initially and some patients are horrified at the thought of introducing a plastic tube into their bodies; however, with motivation, understanding and sensitivity on behalf of the educator, they soon become proficient.

Most people with the right determination can master the technique. Lack of motivation is usually the most common reason for failure. Manual dexterity is essential. A general rule is that if people can write and feed themselves then they usually have the manual dexterity to self-catheterise (Fowler, 1998). Disabilities such as blindness, lack of perineal sensation, tremor, mental disability and paraplegia do not necessarily preclude individuals from being able to master the technique. Where the patient is lacking in manual dexterity a related carer may wish to perform the catheterisation procedure. This is obviously at the request and agreement of the patient (Winder, 1992) and must not be commenced without the carer being educated in the technique and regularly updated.

Every person being taught ISC has different bladder functions and so the regularity of the procedure is dependent on the volume of the residual urine. Frequency of catheterisation must be adhered to as advised. Some patients have to catheterise five or six times a day, others only once a day or week. The aim is to reduce the amount of urine left in the bladder post-voiding or to empty a bladder that is not able to expel urine.

With women, when inserting the catheter, it is essential to experiment with various positions to try to find the one that is the most comfortable and suitable. Some will sit astride a toilet bowl, while others will squat with their backs well supported against a wall with a jug or suitable receptacle on the floor between their legs. Many find that standing with one leg on the edge of the bath is ideal. For men the procedure is much easier. The penis can be held up and out to straighten out the urethra with the catheter held in the other hand (*Figure 7.2*).

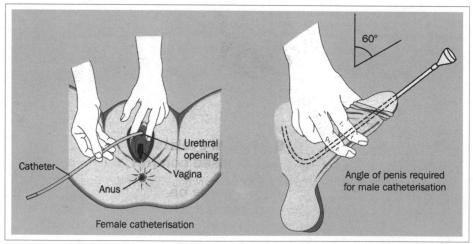

Figure 7.2: When inserting a catheter it is essential that people, particularly women, experiment with various positions to try to find the one that is the most comfortable and suitable for them

The person teaching the technique must monitor how the procedure is carried out, paying special attention to the cleansing of the genital area with soap and water, handwashing, and the correct use of equipment and its disposal. It is human nature to cut corners, but patients must be reminded of the risks associated with this, eg. urinary tract infection or urethral stricture.

Many companies produce literature to support their products; indeed, there are numerous comprehensive booklets on ISC with easy-to-understand points and answers to common questions. It will be difficult for many to grasp all the information on the first visit so it is prudent for the nurse to reassess soon after the initial assessment and to identify any problems such as non-compliance or failure to understand fully the technique.

A high degree of patient satisfaction has been reported by users of the technique (Webb *et al*, 1990).

Advice on when, where, who and how to contact help is desirable and reassuring for the patient. People should not run out of equipment, especially over a holiday period. Prescription services are available throughout the country and are useful for those who, for various reasons such as mobility problems, are unable to access a local pharmacist.

Children at school require a multiprofessional assessment, involving continence advisers, school nurses, teaching staff, occupational therapists or physiotherapists, to develop individualised care plans.

The advantages of intermittent self-catheterisation

ISC offers people an ideal opportunity to become self-caring. Intermittent catheters are less of a risk to health than an indwelling catheter as the latter can cause urethral trauma, urinary tract infection and catheter encrustation (Getliffe and Dolman, 1997). Also, with intermittent catheterisation there is less demand for various pieces of equipment such as drainage bags, spare catheters in case one blocks, and bladder washout solutions to address blockage problems. More importantly, the upper urinary tract is protected from reflux.

Patients with indwelling catheters have great difficulty or find it nearly impossible to express their sexuality without first removing the catheter. With intermittent catheters this is not a problem and sexual intercourse can be spontaneous. The ability to remain sexually active promotes well-being and a positive body image (Winder *et al*, 1997).

In addition, patients involved in planning their own care take more responsibility for that care and, in the long-term, require less nursing intervention.

Catheter selection

Over the past five years several companies have developed single-use sterile catheters and many are now available on prescription. Most of these are made of

PVC and some have a hydrophilic coating (*Table 7.1*). It is advisable to have a hydrophilic coating as there is evidence of stricture formation with long-term 'dry' catheterisation. Where urethral bleeding is present, not allowing the bladder to fill above 450ml can solve the problem. Atonic or non-functioning bladders holding large capacities of urine can become overstretched when pressure builds up. To compensate, the surface area capillaries become larger. When the bladder is emptied artificially the capillaries do not constrict easily which can lead to bleeding.

Table 7.1: Companies that produce intermittent catheters			
Type	**Company**	**Product**	**Address and telephone**
Male and female	Astra Tech	LoFric range	Astra Tech Ltd, Stroudwater Business Park, Brunel Way, Stonehouse, Glos GL10 3SW. Tel: 01453 791763
	Bard	Reliacath	Bard Ltd, Forest House, Brighton Road, Crawley, West Sussex RH11 9BP. Tel: 01293 527888
	Coloplast	EasiCath range Speedicath range	Coloplast Ltd, Peterborough Business Park, Peterborough PE2 6FX. Tel: 01733 392000. Freephone 0800 220622
	Maersk	Puricat range	Maersk Medical Ltd, Thornhill Road, North Moons Moat, Redditch, Worcs B98 9NL. Tel: 01527 64222
	Pennine	O'Neil Intro-Uri-Cath Pre-Lube Nelaton Tiemann	Pennine Healthcare, Newmarket Drive, Ascot Drive Industrial Estate, Derby DE24 8SW. Tel: 01332 571111
	Rüsch	Nelaton Jaques Riplex	Rüsch UK Ltd, Halifax Road, Cressex Business Park, High Wycombe, Bucks HP12 3ST. Tel: 01494 532761
	SIMS Portex	Silky range	SIMS Portex Ltd, Boundary Road, Hythe, Kent CT21 6JL. Tel: 01303 260551
Paediatric	Astra Tech	LoFric paediatric	See above
	Bard	Reliacath	See above
	Coloplast	EasiCath range	See above
	Maersk	Puricat range	See above
	Pennine	Paediatric Nelaton	See above
	Rüsch	Riplex Nelaton Jaques	See above

Informed choice

It is advisable that patients are allowed to decide, having been presented with all the up-to-date information, on the catheter that best suits their needs. Indeed, in many cases the nurse's choice may not be the same as the patient's. There are many good catheters available and patients need to experiment before deciding which is appropriate for them.

Selection of a catheter is very much a personal decision and issues such as life style, work environment, access to toilet facilities, travelling and holidays all need to be considered. The frequency of catheterisation must be discussed and continued as agreed. A list of dos and don'ts is useful as a reminder for patients (*Table 7.2*).

Table 7.2: Dos and don'ts of intermittent catheterisation	
Dos	Eat a well balanced diet to avoid constipation
	Drink 8–10 drinks daily avoiding caffeine
	Pay particular attention to hygiene, ie. handwashing and genitalia
	Use single-use catheters if advised (do not try to reuse)
	Wash reusable catheters carefully and store in an airtight box, dispose of after three days
	Report any changes in urine, ie. blood discolouration, sediment and smell
	Try to pass urine after sexual activity
	Ensure you see your consultant as regularly as appropriate
Don'ts	Catheterise more frequently than advised
	Reuse single-use catheters
	Push if a catheter will not go in easily, try again later
	Pull if a catheter does not come out easily; if this situation occurs, relax, wait 5–10 minutes, then try again
	Give equipment to anyone else
	Run short of catheters, especially over holiday periods
	Take shortcuts with hygiene, infections are common

It is essential that patients performing ISC have follow-up appointments with their consultants and, if appropriate, have upper tract imaging (ultrasound imaging of the kidneys and ureters) to identify any damage to this area which could mean having to perform ISC more frequently. In some areas upper tract imaging is offered to patients on a yearly basis.

Clinical effectiveness

When nurses and patients work together to formulate a plan of care, they must identify the correct package of care for the patient. The goal is to provide care that will cure or manage the patient's condition, and improve the patient's quality of life. In relation to ISC, healthcare professionals must be aware of the most recent research-based literature in order to develop effective standards, guidelines or protocols for good practice (Department of Health, 1998). There are several computer indexes available in health service libraries to enable those involved in health care to search for the most up-to-date information (*Table 7.3*).

Table 7.3: Examples of computer indexes
CINAHL is a nursing and allied health computerised database that includes nursing, health education, occupational therapy and other related publications
British Nursing Index is a nursing database of all British and other major journals that are available in printed form, on computer disks (CD ROMs) and through the Internet
The Cochrane Library is a computerised database that includes the Cochrane Controlled Trials Register, the Cochrane Database of Systematic Reviews, the Database of Abstracts of Reviews of Effectiveness and the Cochrane Review Methodology Database

Conclusion

The clinical effectiveness framework enables nurses to reflect why they do what they do for patients and to find better ways of caring for patients. Clinical effectiveness is about doing the right thing in the right way and at the right time for the right patient (DoH, 1998). ISC empowers patients to take responsibility for their own care. Therefore, the initial time spent teaching and monitoring the patient will bring considerable rewards in the long term.

Patients have the right to be involved in the decision-making process. Nursing is a progressive profession that is able to work in partnership with patients so that health outcomes are improved. Teaching a patient the technique of clean ISC is an example of supporting the patient in order to relinquish some of the care and be satisfied that the care has been effective.

Key points

- ❖ Intermittent self-catheterisation (ISC) is a more appropriate treatment option than indwelling catheters.

- ❖ Extra time spent initially on teaching and monitoring the patient reaps considerable rewards in the long term.

- ❖ ISC enhances patients' quality of life and preserves body image which helps in the continuation of sexual activity.

- ❖ Nurse time is saved by patients taking responsibility for some of their care.

- ❖ Quality of patients' life is promoted by less infections associated with long-term catheters.

References

Brocklehurst JC (1977) The causes and management of incontinence in the elderly. *Nurs Mirror* **144**: 15

Brocklehurst JC, Dillane JB, Griffiths I, Fry J (1968) The prevalence and symptoms of urinary incontinence in an aged population. *Gerontologica Clinica* **10**: 242–53

Chapple C, Christmas T (1990) *Urodynamics Made Easy*. Churchill Livingstone, Edinburgh

Dionko AC, Sondo LP, Hollander JB, Lapides (1985) Fate of patients started on clean intermittent self-catheterisation therapy ten years ago. *J Urol* **129**: 1120–2

DoH (1998) *Achieving Effective Practice. A Cinical Effectiveness and Research Information Pack for Nurses and Health Visitors*. HMSO, London

Fowler CJ (1996) Investigation of the neurogenic bladder. *J Neurol Neurosurg Psychiatry* **60**: 6–13

Fowler CJ (1998) Bladder problems. In: *Multiple Sclerosis Information for Nurses and Health Professionals: Information Pack*. MS Research Trust, Spirella Building, Bridge Road, Letchworth, Herts SG6 4ET

Getliffe K, Dolman M (1997) *Promoting Continence*. Ballière Tindall, London

Guttmann L, Frankel H (1966) The value of intermittent catheterisation in early management of traumatic paraplegia and tetraplegia. *Paraplegia* **4**: 63–84

Herr WH (1975) Intermittent catheterisation in neurogenic bladder dysfunction. *J Urol* **113**: 477–9

Hilton P (1987) Urinary incontinence in women. *Br Med J* **295**: 424–32

Horowitz M, Kuhr CS, Mitchell ME (1995) The Mitrofanoff catheterisable channel: patient acceptance. *J Urol* **153**: 771–2

Lapides J, Ananias CD, Silber SJ, Lowe BS (1972) Clean intermittent self-catheterisation in the treatment of urinary tract disease. *J Urol* **107**: 458–61

Lapides J, Dionko AC, Gould FR (1976) Further observations on self catheterisation. *J Urol* **116**: 169–71

Murray K, Lewis P, Blannin J, Shepherd A (1984) Clean intermittent self-catheterisation in the management of adult lower urinary tract dysfunction. *Br J Urol* **56**: 379–8

Perkash I (1975) Intermittent catheterisation and bladder rehabilitation in the spinal cord injury patient. *J Urol* **114**: 230–3

Sumfest JM, Burns MW, Mitchell ME (1993) The Mitrofanoff principle in urinary reconstruction. *J Urol* **150**: 1875–7

Webb RJ, Lawson AL, Neal DE (1990) Clean intermittent self catheterisation in 172 adults. *Br J Urol* **65**: 20–3

Winder A (1992) Intermittent catheterisation. In: Roe BH, ed. *Clinical Nursing Practice. The Promotion and Management of Incontinence*. 1nt edn. Prentice Hall, London: 157–76

Winder A, Doherty W, Bennett P, Buckley R (1997) *Teaching to Teach Intermittent Self-Catheterisation*. Coloplast, Peterborough

8

Patient management following suprapubic catheterisation

Ian Peate

This chapter considers the issue of suprapubic catheterisation and the subsequent care of the client. The conditions and situations where suprapubic catheterisation may be used are outlined. A review of the literature on this important subject suggests that there is little research/ evidence-based practice to support some current-day practices. The review addresses such issues as what suprapubic catheterisation is and how it is carried out. Key issues such as avoidance of infection, the need for dressings and care of the insertion site are discussed. In particular, the gynaecological field is explored to highlight concern about variations and discrepancies in approaches to care of the patient with a suprapubic catheter *in situ*. Finally, a call is made for practitioners to base their care on research findings or evidence-based practice rather than tradition, ritual or heresy.

This chapter presents a critical analysis of the care and management of a patient with a suprapubic catheter *in situ*. The available literature on the subject is reviewed and current practice is discussed. Ways in which care and management could be improved are suggested, together with recommendations as to how these findings can be disseminated to the healthcare professions.

It is not the author's intention to judge the practice of other professionals in relation to this subject. Clearly, the role of each member of the multidisciplinary team may have a different emphasis and the rationale for this may be based on the perspective taken.

For some time now, it has been fairly widely accepted that, whenever possible, care should be holistic, ie. planned and managed with the underlying principle of recognition of the 'whole' person, embracing the physical, emotional/ psychological, social and spiritual elements of care.

There is concern that, in the past, attention may not always have been given to the overall implications of the use of suprapubic catheterisation. Consequently, the question is raised as to whether all professionals should re-examine their practice in this respect.

Particular concern is expressed over the significant shortage of information on this topic in the nursing literature. There is evidence that nurses may wish to draw on the literature from other disciplines, mainly medicine. It is suggested that nurses may like to review their role and practice in the whole area of urinary catheterisation.

What is suprapubic catheterisation?

Suprapubic catheterisation is performed for a variety of reasons. The care and management of clients with a catheter *in situ* can take place in both community and institutional settings (Winder, 1994). *Table 8.1* lists situations in which suprapubic catheterisation may be indicated.

Table 8.1. Indications for suprapubic catheterisation
Urethral trauma
Clients who require long-term catheterisation and who are sexually active
Following pelvic or urological surgery
Some gynaecological conditions, eg. colposuspension
Long-term catheterisation for incontinence
Clients who are unable to tolerate urethral catheterisation
Some wheelchair-bound clients

Suprapubic catheterisation is an alternative method of urinary diversion, the other being urethral catheterisation. It is also the preferred route of catheterisation for people who are wheelchair users and who may be sexually active and for those who experience difficulties with a urethral catheter.

Despite the wide range of client groups who may require suprapubic catheterisation, there is a dearth of nursing literature relating to the care and management of clients with this type of catheter *in situ*.

This deficiency of information is of concern when the aims of care and management of the patient with an indwelling suprapubic catheter are to maintain comfort, reduce the risk of catheter-associated infection, and to educate carers and clients (Roper *et al*, 1996). In contrast, urethral catheterisation, has received much attention.

Crow *et al* (1988) and Conti and Eutropius (1987) discuss, among other things, cleaning of the urinary meatus. They conclude that the most appropriate and effective way of protecting the urethral meatus is to clean it with soap and water rather than antiseptic lotion. Cleaning of the urethral meatus is not the only important aspect of care — it is just one example of research/evidence-based practice concerning urethral catheterisation. Other considerations, such as the choice of catheter, eg. silicone or latex, the type of drainage system to be used and the client's general condition, are also important.

How is the procedure carried out?

Suprapubic catheterisation involves the insertion of a catheter through the abdominal wall, above the symphysis pubis (suprapubic) into the urinary bladder (*Figure 8.1*). The insertion of a suprapubic catheter is usually undertaken by a medical practitioner, but could be undertaken by the nurse if the nurse is deemed competent, has undertaken a period of extended education and adheres to the guidelines laid down by the UKCC (1992a) in the *Scope of Professional Practice*.

The procedure is performed under local or general anaesthetic, under strict aseptic conditions. Once *in situ*, the catheter is anchored in place either by sutures or by a commercially produced seal and, in some instances, a water-filled balloon. This procedure is different from the insertion of a urethral catheter, which is passed into the urinary bladder via the urethra, with an inflated balloon holding the catheter in place. *Figure 8.2* shows the position of a urethral catheter *in situ* with the balloon inflated. Both systems are connected to a closed drainage system.

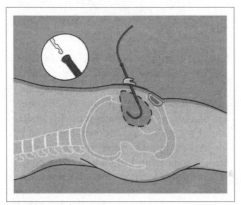
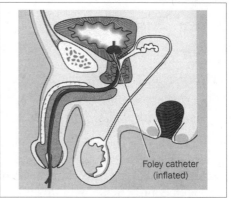

Figure 8.1: Insertion of a catheter above the symphysis pubis (suprapubic). Adapted from Brunner & and Suddarth (1990)

Figure 8.2: Diagrammatic representation of a urethral catheter with the balloon inflated. Adapted from Long *et al* (1996)

The danger of infection

Poor care of the patient with an indwelling suprapubic or urethral catheter, either during the insertion or in the consequent management, can result in dire consequences for the client, both psychologically and physically. Bacteriuria may lead to bacteraemia if a poor technique is used and is associated with significant discomfort and pain. Ascending infection may lead to pyelonephritis and septicaemia.

Prevention of potential infection is the primary aim of care for the patient with a suprapubic catheter *in situ*. Strict aseptic technique must be adhered to when caring for the patient and his/her suprapubic catheter. Long *et al* (1996) suggest that the patient should be encouraged to drink at least 3000ml of fluid per day (unless contraindicated) in order to maintain an adequate urinary output, thus encouraging drainage and reducing the risk of urinary tract infection.

Psychological aspects of suprapubic catheterisation

Patients' perceptions concerning their body image can greatly influence their interpersonal relationships and behaviours. These can be both negative and positive influences. Sundeen *et al* (1994) point out that how a person feels about him/herself is related to how he/she feels about his/her body. The body is a dynamic and continually changing entity and modifications are occurring constantly, both physically and psychologically. The insertion of a suprapubic catheter can be seen as one of these modifications and the perceptions are both physical and psychological.

Self-esteem is a personality variable that can be affected by altered body image. Problems may arise when the individual's self-concept does not meet with notions of his/her own self-ideal, and low self-regard or low self-esteem may result (Sundeen *et al*, 1994). It is important to encourage the client to voice fears and anxieties regarding altered body image. Thus, the nurse must consider the patient from a holistic perspective. Clients may have many other fears, eg. loss of 'normal' body function, potential smell/odour, leakage, visibility of drainage bag, the outcome of having to tell a new sexual partner, and what the client needs to do with the appliance during sexual activity.

Long *et al* (1996) suggest that the nurse can promote a positive body image by offering reassurance (positive regard), encouragement and specific information regarding the management of the suprapubic catheter. Emphasis must be placed on the activities that the patient can do and those that are within his/her control. Realistic aims must be stated in order to encourage the patient to be positive about his/her image.

Suprapubic catheterisation in gynaecology

Some gynaecological conditions such as colposuspension are seen as a valid reason for the intraoperative insertion of a suprapubic catheter. Indeed, Stanton (1992) states that approximately 50% of patients will develop urinary retention following an anterior repair; consequently, many gynaecologists now use suprapubic catheterisation as a preventative measure. Hilton and Stanton (1983) discuss the use of colposuspension for genuine stress incontinence and the insertion of a suprapubic catheter postoperatively to allow adequate urinary drainage.

Colposuspension is a procedure that is used to help to correct urinary incontinence. Gould (1990) refers to this as a 'repair operation'. An incision is made in the vagina and the vesicovaginal fascia is then sutured tightly. The operative site often becomes oedematous; if this involves the urethra, it may lead to micturition problems postoperatively. A suprapubic catheter is therefore inserted during surgery in order to prevent retention of urine and further trauma to the oedematous urethra. The passage of a urethral catheter through an oedematous urethra may be difficult or impossible.

Telephone enquiries to ten hospitals revealed that subsequent care and management regarding the clamping of the suprapubic catheter and the length of time it remained *in situ* varied from hospital to hospital. In some instances, the catheter stayed *in situ* for two days postoperatively and in others up to five days postoperatively.

Mattingly *et al* (1972) demonstrated that suprapubic catheterisation in post-gynaecological conditions resulted in less bacterial infection of the urinary bladder than did urethral catheterisation. Suprapubic catheterisation also reduced the length of hospitalisation. Shute and MacKinnon (1970) investigated how best to manage the postoperative gynaecological client and suggest the use of suprapubic catheters as opposed to urethral catheters in the attempt to reduce genito-urinary tract infection rates.

An holistic approach

Generally, the medical system has focused on the manifestations of illness. In holistic health care the person is encouraged to demonstrate his/her potential as a unique and dynamic person (Sundeen *et al*, 1994). Nurses are able to encourage this potential in individuals. Nursing is primarily concerned with assisting individuals to achieve the best possible state of health that is appropriate for that individual. This state of health will promote the highest level of achievement that that person is able to achieve.

According to Heath (1995), nurses help patients to regain health through the healing process. The healing process in this respect is not only related to curing a specific disease; when considering the patient with an indwelling suprapubic catheter the nurse must address issues that encompass the whole person, ie. holistic care, which includes taking steps to restore emotional and social well-being.

All of the above studies have focused on the 'management' of the suprapubic catheter and were undertaken by colleagues in the medical field. As previously stated, attempts to locate information within the literature regarding the nursing care and management of individuals with a suprapubic catheter *in situ* revealed very little indeed.

Winder's (1994) paper is a community-focused discussion and demonstrates ways in which district nurses can competently 'manage clients' with suprapubic catheters. Again, the focus of the paper is prevention of infection. Other important nursing considerations, such as altered body image and the psychological impact that a suprapubic catheter may have on an individual, are often omitted. It is evident that there is a void in the nursing literature regarding the nursing care and nursing management of clients with suprapubic catheters *in situ*. There may be a variety of reasons for this, but I would suggest that one reason is that urethral catheters and suprapubic catheters are often, mistakenly, thought to be one and the same thing. Indeed, Winder (1994) comments:

The management of urethral and suprapubic catheters is the same; the same types of drainage bags can be used and the same instructions given to patients.

Sturevant-Clinton and Berding (1992) also make the same mistake:

Care of the patient with suprapubic drainage is similar to care of the patient with continuous urethral catheter drainage.

The care of the patient with a suprapubic catheter *in situ* is outlined below.

Care of the suprapubic catheter

Although the principle of care and management of the suprapubic catheter are similar to those of the care and management of a urethral catheter, there are differences.

The suprapubic catheter emerges at right angles to the abdomen and needs to be supported in this position. The activities of personal hygiene and dressing are also compromised to a greater extent with a suprapubic catheter than with a urethral catheter.

The suprapubic catheter is often secured with tape and other dressings; these provide ideal conditions for colonisation by pathogenic bacteria. Dressings and tapes should only be used sparingly when absolutely necessary — enough to secure the catheter. If dressings are to be used, they must be sterile and applied using an aseptic technique. Wilson (1995) points out that there is much conflicting evidence about the most effective type of dressing to be used, and suggests that the type of dressing selected should depend on the specific needs and conditions of the patient.

Unfortunately, Winder (1994) recommends that 'the entry site should be inspected daily and cleaned with antispetic...' This recommendation, however, is not based on sound scientific evidence. The practice of taking dressings down to inspect wounds on a daily basis has long since ceased (the insertion of a suprapubic catheter is a surgical procedure and thus strict asepsis must be maintained during all subsequent care and management of the catheter, as with all surgical incisions). Wilson (1995) recommends that the dressing should be left undisturbed unless there is evidence to suggest otherwise.

Thomlinson (1987) discusses this in some detail. The use of an antiseptic lotion to cleanse a wound, in this case the sutures anchoring the device to the abdominal wall, is contraindicated. Brennan *et al* (1984) condemn the use of antiseptics on wounds: when antiseptics such as chlorhexidine gluconate or povidone iodine are used the blood flow to the site may be adversely affected and lead to poor wound healing. Hence, it would appear that while daily wound inspection and the use of antiseptics to cleanse wounds have ceased in other areas of surgical care, practice in relation to the insertion site of the suprapubic catheter needs reviewing and updating.

Clients with suprapubic catheters *in situ* in their own home will need detailed advice/information regarding wound cleansing and appropriate dressings. Wilson (1995) considers the management of intravesicular devices at home. Similar tailor-made advice is also applicable to the patient who is living at home with a suprapubic catheter *in situ*. Wilson suggests that it is important to keep the plan of care simple, as much distress can be caused by overburdening the patient with unfamiliar procedures. She insists, however, that the general principles of infection control are adhered to.

The literature (eg. Winder, 1994) has indicated that inappropriate practice may still be occurring. The potentially high risk of bacteraemia, resulting from bacteriuria induced by poor, ill-informed care, could lead to serious complications. It is in the care of women undergoing gynaecological surgery that almost all of the ambiguity remains, as many women undergoing gynaecological procedures involving the vagina, uterus and urethra often have suprapubic catheters *in situ*. *Figure 8.3* outlines the factors to consider when deciding whether to perform suprapubic or urethral catheterisation.

Consider suprapubic or urethral catheterisation	
Suprapubic	**Urethral**
Long-term (including incontinence)	Short-term
Sexually active clients	Intermittent
Post-specific surgery	Post-specific surgery
Urethral trauma	Difficulties with suprapubic
Some wheelchair-bound clients	
Difficulties with urethral catheter	
Specific care	
Strict asepsis on insertion	Strict asepsis on insertion
Strict asepsis when cleaning	
Specific advantages	
Reduced risk of infection	Nurse able to carry out procedure;
Enables sexual intercourse	therefore, care will be client directed from the point of insertion
Specific disadvantages	
Altered body image	Altered body image
Potential leakage from and around site	Impedes sexual intercourse
Limited nursing research surrounding the subject	Higher risk of infection
Often requires a registered medical practitioner to insert	

Figure 8.3: Factors to consider when deciding whether to perform suprapubic or urethral catheterisation

Accountability and evidence-based practice

There may be a variety of reasons why ambiguity surrounding the care of the patient with a suprapubic catheter *in situ* persists. Anecdotal evidence in the gynaecological setting suggests that the management of the suprapubic catheter has become the immediate responsibility of the gynaecologist, who ultimately determines the length of time the catheter stays *in situ* and the ritual surrounding the clamping of the catheter. This can prove problematic in practice. Where there is more than one gynaecologist, a conflict of opinion and interest may arise. Nurses working in the clinical area may have to care for and manage patients who are the clients of different gynaecologists. This conflict can cause concern for both client and nurse.

It could be suggested that these various methods (eg. the length of time a catheter remains *in situ* and clamping the catheter) are not based on any single, valid and reliable piece of empirical work. When asked, the ten hospitals surveyed over the telephone replied that the catheter stayed *in situ* according to the gynaecologist's preference; there was no evidence explicitly known to the respondent to support the practice. Hence the gynaecologist's preference could conflict with the unique individual needs of each client. Review of the medical literature revealed that much of the practice draws upon the biological sciences. The psychological aspects of care appear to have been glossed over.

If these propositions are true — and anecdotal evidence and the dearth of nursing literature on this issue would appear to confirm this — then nurses caring for women with suprapubic catheters *in situ* are in some way contravening their Code of Professional Conduct (UKCC, 1992b) which requires them to:

> *... safeguard and promote the interests of individual patients and clients.*

However, clause six states that nurses must:

> *... work in a collaborative and co-operative manner with healthcare professionals and others involved in providing care, and recognise and respect their particular contributions within the care team.*

It must be emphasised that the Code expressly states that nurses must work in a collaborative manner with others and not in a collusive manner. While it is essential that each individual should recognise the contribution of others involved in the care of any one patient, it must also be remembered that patients have rights too.

Dispelling ritual — putting the client first

Nurses working with, and caring for, individuals with suprapubic catheters *in situ* must base their care on sound principles. It is suggested, therefore, that they should use nursing research, relevant knowledge, attitudes and skills in management and care of individuals with indwelling suprapubic catheters to enhance comfort, prevent both psychological and physiological complications, and enhance the clients' quality of life.

If care is based on a sound research/evidence base, then the client's overall satisfaction with his/her care may be enhanced. Thus the edicts of The Patient's Charter (Department of Health, 1991) will not be empty political rhetoric but a true attempt to improve standards of care. It is conceded, however, that the paucity of nursing literature surrounding the subject area may initially make this objective difficult to achieve. However, nurses must question current practice, reflect on their actions (Atkins and Murphy, 1995) and thus begin to influence care by further qualitative and quantitative analysis.

Hunt (1987) suggests several reasons why variations in nursing practice may occur, eg. the autonomy exercised by the ward sister and the problems associated with change strategies. Hunt's comments go some way to suggesting that there is a power differential at work when attempting to change practice. I would suggest that this power differential in the case of the care and management of the woman with a suprapubic catheter *in situ* following a gynaecological procedure (eg. colposuspension) is dominated by the gynaecologist and medicine.

Standard setting

There are ways in which some of these inconsistencies in care can be remedied or at best acknowledged. In certain areas of care, eg. oral hygiene, the care and management of individuals requiring this form of intervention are based on sound theoretical knowledge. The aim, therefore, is to focus on the knowledge, experiences and expertise of the multidisciplinary team in order to set standards to improve the provision of care for people with suprapubic catheters *in situ*. However, although this may appear to be the panacea for all ills associated with suprapubic catheterisation, it is not.

There can be no universal approach to the care and management of the individual with a suprapubic catheter *in situ*, or any other problem. However, evidence-based guidelines may go some way to ensuring that the best possible care is given. Each individual is a unique being. It must also be remembered that each registered nurse is accountable to the patient for his/her practice. The use of standard setting, according to Hunt (1987), is one way of achieving such accountability.

Conclusion

This chapter has demonstrated a paucity of nursing research relating to the care and management of the individual with a suprapubic catheter *in situ*. Much of the literature reviewed had a strong medical bias and tended to concentrate on the physiological aspects of care. Through systematic nursing enquiry (nursing research), nurses need to consider the psychological as well as the physical aspects associated with suprapubic catheterisation.

Nurses are in an ideal position to take the care and management of patients undergoing suprapubic catheterisation forward in order to meet the specific needs of the patient as opposed to tradition. It is suggested that nurses may be encouraged (with sufficient support) to lead the way concerning the insertion of suprapubic catheters, as is the case with urethral catheters.

Examination of the conditions and situations that necessitate the insertion of a suprapubic catheter, particularly gynaecological procedures, revealed a tremendous variation in association with practices, such as wound care and cleansing and the management of the catheter post-colposuspension. Concern arose regarding the nurse's role in these practices.

It is suggested that nurses need to adopt a multidisciplinary approach, in order to set standards regarding the care of individuals with a suprapubic catheter *in situ*. This would hopefully result in providing the client with the most appropriate care, which embraces both the psychological and physiological aspects. Such an approach may enable nurses to increase their knowledge base, with a high emphasis on the holistic perspective.

A small-scale study is being planned in order to investigate this issue further. This study aims to describe the care delivered to a small sample of women who have undergone colposuspension which necessitated the insertion of a suprapubic catheter.

Key points

❖ Aspects of suprapubic catheterisation and the appropriate associated care are, in some instances, in a state of confusion.

❖ Suprapubic catheterisation and urethral catheterisation are different procedures and their care and management require different approaches.

❖ Nurses must base their care of the patient with a suprapubic catheter *in situ* on sound evidence and not tradition, ritual and hearsay.

❖ In order to address this important issue, enhance care and add to the body of knowledge, a multidisciplinary approach is advocated, possibly in the form of standard setting.

References

Atkins S, Murphy K (1995) Reflective practice. *Nurs Standard* **9**(45): 31–5

Brennan SS, Foster ME, Leaper DJ (1984) Adverse effects of antiseptics on the healing process. *J Hosp Infect* **5**: 122

Brunner LS, Suddarth DS (1990) *The Lippincott Manual of Medical-Surgical Nursing*. 2nd edn. Harper and Row, London

Conti MT, Eutropius L (1987) Preventing urinary tract infection — what really works? *Am J Nurs* **87**: 307–9

Crow R, Mulhall A, Chapman R (1988) Indwelling catheterisation and related nursing practice. *J Adv Nurs* **13**: 489–95

Department of Health (1991) *The Patient's Charter.* HMSO, London

Gould D (1990) *Nursing Care of Women.* Prentice Hall, London

Heath HB (1995) *Foundations in Nursing Theory and Practice.* Mosby, London

Hilton P, Stanton SL (1983) A clinical and urodynamic assessment of the Burch colposuspension for genuine stress incontinence. *Br J Obstet Gynaecol* **90**: 934–9

Hunt M (1987) The process of translating research findings into nursing practice. *J Adv Nurs* **12**: 101–10

Long BC, Phipps WJ, Cassmeyer VJ (1996) *Adult Nursing: A Nursing Process Approach.* Mosby, London

Mattingly R, Moore D, Clark D (1972) Bacteriologic study of suprapubic bladder drainage. *Am J Obstet Gynecol* **114**: 732–8

Roper N, Logan W, Tierney A (1996) *The Elements of Nursing: A model for nursing based on a model of living.* 4th edn. Churchill Livingstone, Edinburgh

Shute WB, MacKinnon KJ (1970) Postoperative restoration of micturition with suprapubic catheterisation. *Am J Obstet Gynaecol* **106**: 943–6

Stanton SL (1992) Vaginal prolapse. In: Shaw R, Soutter P, Stanton S eds. *Gynaecology.* Churchill Livingstone, Edinburgh: 437–47

Sturevant-Clinton DR, Berding C (1992) Disorders of the ureters, bladder and urethra. In: Burrel LO, ed. *Adult Nursing in Hospital and Community Settings.* Appleton and Lange, Norwalk: 1288–308

Sundeen SJ, Stuart GW, Rankin EA, Cohen SA (1994) *Nurse-Client Interaction.* 5th edn. Mosby, St Louis

Thomlinson D (1987) To clean or not to clean? *Nurs Times* **83**(37): 71–85

UKCC (1992A) *The Scope of Professional Practice.* UKCC, London

UKCC (1992b) *Code of Professional Conduct for the Nurse, Midwife and Health Visitor.* UKCC, London

Wilson J (1995) *Infection Control in Clinical Practice.* Baillière Tindall, London

Winder A (1994) Suprapubic catheterisation. *Comm Outlook* **4**(12): 25–6

Section three
Minimising and troubleshooting
common catheter problems

9

Troubleshooting common problems associated with long-term urinary catheters

Margaret Rew, Sue Woodward

A catheter complications survey study, carried out over a two-year period in three Bristol health districts, recorded 506 emergency referrals during a six-month period (Kohler-Ockmore and Feneley, 1996). A further detailed study on 54 of the patients showed that 48% experienced catheter blockage and 37% reported urine bypassing. Urinary catheterisation can cause many health problems; bacteriuria is inevitable in long-term catheterised patients (Cravens and Zweig, 2000). This chapter identifies some of the common problems that can occur with long-term catheters, makes recommendations and applies an evidence-based approach to catheter care. In order to identify and treat the associated problems, it is necessary to understand the anatomy and functions of the bladder. The chapter addresses this before examining the problems, which include: catheter blockage; bypassing of urine; catheter rejection and balloon non-deflation; and latex allergy. The psychological and social aspects, although not covered in this chapter, are also important and should always be considered along with all other aspects of care.

Up to 12.6% of hospitalised patients and 4% of community patients have urethral catheters (Crow *et al*, 1986). The management of long-term catheters is a subject of constant debate. Although continence awareness is increasing all the time and hopefully patients are properly assessed before a decision is reached regarding the management of their incontinence, urinary catheters still remain a common feature in patients' long-term care.

Many people with intractable incontinence find that catheterisation enhances their quality of life (Nazarko, 1998). However, the practice of catheterising patients to manage their continence problem sometimes causes more problems than it solves.

Urinary catheterisation is a common procedure which can take the form of either intermittent catheterisation or indwelling/self-retaining catheterisation. The two routes of inserting the indwelling catheter are urethral and suprapubic. This latter method sees the catheter being inserted through the abdominal wall above the symphysis pubis, and has been advocated for patients with neuropathic bladder dysfunction or following complications of urethral catheterisation. It may also be more appropriate than the urethal catheter for those patients who are wheelchair bound, as they may find it easier to clean and change, and those who are sexually active.

Whether the method used is urethral or suprapubic, many of the problems that occur are the same. The two major differences are the absence of urethral trauma and an association with lower infection rates with suprapubic catheters, although with prolonged drainage, infection is almost inevitable (Winder, 1994).

According to Getliffe and Dolman (1997), the main aims of catheter management are as listed in *Table 9.1*. The skills and knowledge needed to achieve these are complex and require an holistic approach with ongoing assessment of the patient, taking into account all the constantly changing influences and circumstances of their needs.

In understanding how to manage complications with long-term catheters it is important to be first familiar with the basic anatomy and physiology of the urinary system (*Figure 9.1*).

Table 9.1: The main aims of catheter management
To relieve and manage urinary dysfunction
To recognise and minimise risks of secondary complications
To promote patient dignity and comfort and to assist patients to reach their own potential in terms of self-care and independence
To provide a cost-effective service
Source: Getliffe and Dolman (1997)

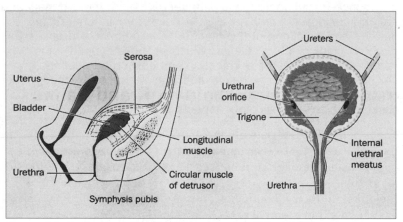

Figure 9.1: A diagram showing the anatomy of the bladder

Anatomy

The bladder is situated in the pelvis behind the symphysis pubis and in front of the rectum. In women, it lies in front of the uterus. The bladder acts as a storage reservoir for urine. Urine is transported from the kidneys to the bladder by the ureters, which are made of peristaltic muscle, and which enter the bladder near its base in the small triangular area known as the trigone. The ureters run obliquely through the bladder wall for about 1.5cm to open into the bladder at the left and right ureteric orifices. The third point of the trigone is formed by the internal urethral meatus.

The trigone contains a large number of sensory nerve endings which are very sensitive to stretch. When pressure inside the bladder increases during filling, the function of the trigone is to prevent reflux of urine by compressing the ureters. Impulses are sent to the spinal cord and on to the brain, via the pelvic nerves, as the bladder fills. This triggers messages to be sent back along the same route, causing the detrusor muscle to contract and the urethal sphincter mechanism to relax, thus allowing the person to pass urine.

The bladder wall comprises four layers: the innermost mucosal layer; the submucosa made of connective tissue; the detrusor muscle consisting of layers of circular and longitudinal muscle fibres; and the outermost layer, the serosa, which is composed of peritoneum and covers only the upper surface of the bladder. When the detrusor muscle contracts it causes the bladder to reduce in length and diameter so that it is emptied effectively.

Control over the micturition process allows the person to delay going to the toilet, and anything that interrupts the process, eg. neurological disease, detrusor instability or congenital abnormalities, will lead to continence problems. Similarly when examining catheter problems it is often detrusor instability or trigone irritation that is the cause of the problem.

Catheter problems

Bypassing

Bypassing, when urine leaks around the catheter, occurs at some time in up to 89% of patients with a long-term catheter (Roe and Brocklehurst, 1987). This causes much distress and embarrassment to the patient, and can hinder the accurate monitoring of urine output. The most common causes of bypassing are listed in *Table 9.2*.

Constipation: Constipation may develop as a result of a variety of factors, eg. diet and fluid intake and the overuse of laxatives, which can exacerbate constipation by causing colonic damage (Read *et al*, 1995).

In relation to catheter care, constipation can cause pressure on the drainage lumen and prevent the catheter from draining (Rigby, 1998). If constipation is suspected, an examination is required and the appropriate treatment given.

Table 9.2: Common causes of bypassing
Constipation
Kinked tubing
Catheter size and length/balloons
Detrusor instability
Trigone irriation
Blockage

An adequate intake of fluid and fibre is an important part of a healthy diet and could reduce the occurrence of laxative overuse. The general recommendation for the minimum amount of fluid intake to maintain good health is 1.5 litres/day (Addison, 1997), but this must take into account an individual's body weight and any specific fluid requirements. For example, if the patient is pyrexial he/she may need extra fluids; similarly, a person with constipation may require extra fluids as this may prevent constipation (Bush, 2000).

Kinked tubing: If the catheter or the drainage tubing becomes kinked or compressed this will cause occlusion and the urine, being unable to drain freely, will build up and may bypass around the catheter. Kinked tubing also may lead to an increased infection risk to the patient (Godfrey and Evans, 2000).

All that may be required to avoid this is to reposition the patient, catheter or tubing. The drainage bag should be placed lower than the level of the bladder to allow the urine to drain properly. However, it has been shown that if the drainage bag is hung too low below the bladder a suction, or negative pressure, occurs within the catheter, drawing the bladder mucosa up against the eyes of the catheter, thus causing blockage (Lowthian, 1998).

Catheters can easily become kinked if attention is not paid to using the correct size and length.

Catheter size and length/balloons: A catheter of appropriate length should be selected, as excess catheter can result in loss of dignity and increase risk of trauma or blockage as a result of kinking (Godfrey and Evans, 2000) (*Figure 9.2*).

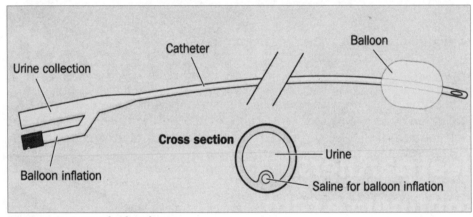

Figure 9.2: A standard catheter

The selection process should take into account the patient's lifestyle, gender and mobility. Catheters come in different lengths: standard, paediatric and female. Variations sometimes occur dependent upon the material, eg. some 100% silicone catheters are longer than some latex catheters. Generally, the standard or male length catheter is between 40cm and 44cm long and the female catheter is 26cm. Female catheters should be used for females where possible as the reduced length outside the body results in less 'pulling' on the catheter. However, if the patient is obese or is wheelchair bound the female length catheter may kink or be uncomfortable and produce pressure reactions around the groin or thigh. For these patients a standard length catheter may be more appropriate.

Catheter size is usually measured in Charrière (Ch) units, which is a measure of the catheter's diameter in millimetres (1 Ch = 0.33mm diameter). The smallest size of catheter that will drain the contents of the bladder should be selected (Norton, 1996). A size of 12–14 Ch is appropriate for a female patient, and 12–16 Ch for a male patient. A size 12 Ch can cope with over 100 litres of urine per day. Larger sizes (more than 16 Ch) are rarely required and are usually used where there is a large amount of blood clots and tissue debris draining via the lumen.

Larger sized catheters can not only cause pain and discomfort, but also irritation, trauma and bypassing. They distend the elastic tissue of the urethral mucosa, so that it is unable to close its natural folds around the catheter thus causing leakage around the sides. Replacing a leaking catheter with a smaller one may reduce the problem. Larger size catheters are also associated with abscess formation and with increased infection risk (Roe and Brocklehurst, 1987).

The balloon size is also important, as large balloons can cause irrigation of the urethral mucosa and trigone of the bladder, which may in turn lead to bladder spasm and bypassing of urine. The balloon must be inflated with the specified amount of sterile water that is recommended by the manufacturers and written on the packaging. Partial, or over-inflation of the balloon causes an asymmetrical balloon, which can deflect the tip and cause irritation to the bladder wall, spasm and possible necrosis.

Detrusor instability and trigone irritation: Normally, the detrusor muscle is relaxed during bladder filling and only contracts when voluntary emptying is initiated. Detrusor instability, or 'unstable bladder', is when the contractions occur spontaneously or as a result of provocations such as coughing or vigorous exercise.

In the uncatheterised patient, the bladder is not emptied properly and the patient may complain of urgency and be incontinent before reaching the toilet. The bladder function decreases as its storing capabilities decrease.

In the catheterised patient, the contractions may be strong enough to cause leakage around the catheter and bladder spasm and the bladder's decreased functional ability adds to the problem.

A smaller size catheter, which causes less irritation, may help. Alternatively, the treatment is to use anticholinergic medications such as oxybutynin or tolterodine. These drugs reduce the muscular spasm of the detrusor by blocking the action of the neurotransmitter, acetylcholine. Care must be taken to monitor for constipation, as these drugs also act on the muscles of the colon resulting in prolonged transit time. For the uncatheterised patient presenting with these symptoms, a bladder retraining programme may be helpful (Anders, 1999).

Trigone irritation can be caused when the balloon is not inflated properly, as mentioned above:

Blockage: If a catheter blocks, bypassing is likely to occur. The blockage could be the result of any of the reasons given above as well as haematuria, debris and encrustation. A good fluid intake helps to 'flush' the catheter through and to dilute concentrated urine or urine with debris/light haematuria. Dilution is also thought to impair bacterial growth, and flushing reduces the likelihood of bacteria ascending from the bag (Wilson, 1997).

One of the most common causes of blockage is the deposit of mineral salts or encrustations on the catheter surface, and it affects about 50% of long-term catheterised patients (Getliffe, 1996). It causes problems that are distressing to the patients and carers and costly in time and resources to the health service.

These encrustations build up following urease activity. Urease is an enzyme produced by bacteria in the urine. It splits urinary urea into ammonia and carbon dioxide and alters the pH balance of the urine to an increase in alkalinity. This leads to the development of crystals, which adhere to the catheter. Bacteria then adhere to the crystals and the cycle continues. Hedelin *et al* (1991) showed that patients with a mean urinary pH below 6.8 had minute traces of encrustation, while patients above pH 6.8 had considerably more.

In the Kohler-Ockmore and Feneley (1996) study, blockage was associated with bladder stones, a high urinary pH and bacteria in the urine. The crystals are of struvite (ammonium magnesium phosphate) and hydroxyapatite (calcium phosphate), and they build up in the catheter lumen, around the eyeholes and the catheter balloon.

No catheter material is resistant to encrustation (Morris *et al*, 1997), although different materials have shown to differ in the rate at which they become encrusted. For example, catheters made of pure latex encrust faster than all-silicone or hydrogel-coated catheters.

Management of catheter encrustation has largely depended on the use of catheter maintenance solutions. However, all aspects of catheter care need to be taken into consideration when planning the management of the catheter. This includes the patient's activity and mobility, diet and fluid intake, hygiene needs, and building up a catheter history upon which to base future care regimes. It has been suggested that between three and five consecutive catheters should be observed in order to establish a clear pattern of catheter history (Norberg *et al*, 1983). The probable cause of the blockage problems can then be diagnosed and an appropriate regime of care planned.

It is important to document the length of time taken between the insertion of the catheter and the catheter becoming blocked. If a catheter becomes blocked, it should be removed and split open to check for encrustation or debris. It is also useful to check the level of the urinary pH regularly so as to monitor change and possibly avoid a blockage problem. If encrustation is identified, the catheter may be changed more frequently to avoid blockage problems (Evans *et al*, 2001). However, if the catheter blocks frequently, the use of a catheter maintenance solution may be preferable to frequent changes. Maintenance solutions are listed in *Table 9.3*.

For their administration, the solution to be used is warmed to body temperature, by immersing the bag in lukewarm water, and the bag is then connected to the catheter using an aseptic technique. The contents should be instilled using the force of gravity (Rew, 1999). The traditional method of using a 50–60ml syringe has been shown to be potentially damaging to the tissues because of the force on the syringe (Getliffe and Dolman, 1997); using gravity and as little pressure as possible is preferable.

Table 9.3: Catheter maintenance solutions
Citric acid 3.23% (Suby G): this is used if the patient is identified as having encrustation blockages. A regular regime can be used to help slow the rate at which the catheter encrusts and blocks. The frequency of use depends on the individual patient and the frequency of blockage. This must be continually monitored as there is always a risk of introducing further infection each time the closed system is disrupted, and it is therefore important to only give solutions when indicated rather than just because the patient has always had them
Citric acid 6% (Solution R): this is used for persistent 'blockers' or when Suby G is ineffective. It may also be used before catheter removal to dissolve crystals that have formed around the tip causing trauma to the delicate urethral tissues
Mandelic acid: this is effective in reducing the colony count of several species of micro-organisms including *Pseudomonas spp.* and *Escherichia coli* (King and Stickler, 1992)
Chlorhexidine (1:500): this should only be used for a short course of treatment, as studies have shown that continuous use does not prevent or eliminate the common infecting organisms and may lead to the development of resistant organisms (King and Stickler, 1992)
Sodium chloride (NaCI 0.9%): this is recommended to flush out debris or mucus. It has purely a mechanical action

There has been some debate recently as to whether 'gentle agitation' is better when instilling these solutions. Getliffe *et al* (2000) state that 'gentle agitation did not significantly improve the dissolution of encrustation'. This research also showed that volumes of 50ml are just as effective as 100ml, being enough to completely fill the catheter lumen and bathe the tip in the solution.

Latex allergy

Latex allergy was first documented in 1979 and there is increasing evidence that the coating on a latex catheter does not necessarily provide protection from the latex (Woodward, 1997). All patients should be screened for latex allergy before catheterisation to assess the degree of risk. If 100% silicone catheters are used, balloon inflation should be checked periodically because these are highly permeable (Winn, 1998).

It is recommended that patients with latex allergy are catheterised with 100% silicone (Woodward, 1997) or silastic catheters (Cravens and Zweig, 2000). This aspect of catheter care has been covered in detail elsewhere (Woodward, 1997).

Catheter rejection

Catheter rejection has received little attention and describes the problem of a patient who apparently pulls out his/her catheter (Belfield, 1985). It may be caused by a variety of reasons. It has been known for a patient to deliberately pull out a urethral catheter, with the balloon inflated. This is usually because of the patient being in a confused state and lacking comprehension about this device.

A urinary catheter may be causing the patient discomfort and irritation, and he/she may attempt to remove that stimulus without realising the implications of their actions. If this is the case it is better to find another way of managing the bladder problem, and for this reason catheter rejection could be considered a contraindication for urethral catheterisation (Rigby, 1998).

If the patient is in urinary retention and bladder drainage is essential, then a suprapubic catheter may cause less irritation, but it is best to avoid catheterisation if at all possible.

A catheter may also be expelled per urethra because of detrusor hyper-reflexia, where the detrusor muscle goes into spasm and contracts in an attempt to expel the catheter. This may be caused by the tip of the catheter irritating the sensitive trigone area of the bladder, as described previously. It may also be caused when a catheterised patient is straining at stool (Rigby, 1998). If detrusor hyper-reflexia is suspected then this can often be successfully treated with an anticholinergic drug.

One study conducted to investigate the nature of catheter rejection concluded that in only one-third of cases the catheter was pulled out. The majority were spontaneously expelled as a result of weak pelvic floor muscles, urethral dilation and detrusor hyper-reflexia. The cause was uncertain in approximately 25% of cases (Belfield, 1985). Whatever the cause, 10% of cases of catheter rejection were associated with significant complications, such as trauma and haematuria, which may lead to urethral stricture (narrowing of the urethra) in the long-term.

It is important that catheter rejection is identified wherever possible and that other means of managing the urinary problem are sought. If catheterisation is essential, then small Ch and balloon sizes should be selected to reduce the motor and sensory irritation caused.

Pain and trauma

Many people experience pain and discomfort, which may not be related to trauma (Winn, 1998). In one study, 39% of patients had some discomfort (Crow *et al*, 1986), and it is a continual problem for 8% of patients (Kennedy *et al*, 1983). Patients often complain of cramping pain, similar to dysmenorrhoea. If this is the case, simple analgesia should be offered. If the pain is persistent, this may be the result of unstable detrusor contractions and should be treated accordingly.

A catheter which is too large may cause trauma to the urethral mucosa and may obstruct paraurethral glands and cause urethritis (Alderman, 1989). Once again this highlights the need for selection of a small balloon, inflated with 10ml of sterile water for injections. Once inserted, the catheter may be anchored to prevent urethral traction and trauma (Cravens and Zweig, 2000).

Urethral pressure ulcers have also been demonstrated following urethral catheterisation, especially at the external sphincter and the penoscrotal junction in men, where the catheter bends. This can lead to the development of urethral strictures (Lowthian, 1995). The catheter tip may also lead to erosion within the bladder and fistulae may result. It has also been shown that long-term use of indwelling catheters may lead to malignancy (Alderman, 1989).

Balloon non-deflation

This problem becomes apparent when attempting to remove a self-retaining catheter and the water cannot be withdrawn from the balloon. The problem of balloon non-deflation has been recognised for a long time and yet has received little attention in the nursing literature. It may occur for a variety of reasons, and a number of possible solutions have been advocated over the years.

One of the most common causes of balloon non-deflation is a physical obstruction which compresses the catheter inflation channel. This may be caused by constipation and faecal impaction or by kinked catheter tubing which prevents the water from exiting the balloon. These problems are easily remedied by removing the obstruction and straightening the tubing, but often these obvious and simple solutions are overlooked.

Balloon non-deflation may also be caused by encrustation around the balloon area, making it difficult to deflate (Britton and Wright, 1990). This may be remedied by using a catheter maintenance solution (Solution R) in an attempt to dissolve the encrustation, but this is not always successful and another method of balloon puncture needs to be employed.

Before resorting to more radical methods of balloon puncture, such as using a transperitoneal approach, there are some very simple techniques that could be tried. First, it may simply be that the syringe used to deflate the balloon is faulty; the syringe should be changed and the procedure attempted again. The syringe should never be drawn forcefully as this may cause a vacuum to be created within the inflation channel, causing it to collapse. The syringe should be left in place for a few minutes to allow the water to drain spontaneously. If this does not work, then a sterile needle should be attached to a 10ml syringe and the needle inserted into the arm of the catheter just above the inflation valve in case it is this that is faulty. The water should be removed gently in this way.

When attempting to remove a catheter with a non-deflating balloon, the catheter should never be cut. If the catheter is under traction it may disappear inside the urethra; also, if the valve has been cut off and the water does not escape from the balloon, then it will no longer be possible to try some of the more simple methods of balloon deflation. In case there is a small particulate obstruction of the inflation channel, it may be useful to insert a further 2ml of sterile water for injection in an attempt to unblock it.

Under no circumstances should an attempt be made to fill the balloon until it bursts inside the bladder. The volumes needed to achieve this are not insignificant and rupture of the balloon in this way has been shown to lead to free fragment formation within the bladder, which may result in further trauma, irritation, and infection (Crisp and Nacey, 1990), or in bladder stone formation (Godwin and Lloyd, 1990).

Many more invasive methods of balloon rupture have been reported if simple solutions are ineffective. The use of mineral oil solvents and ether have been suggested to dissolve the balloon, but this has resulted in cystitis and so is no longer advocated (Wilde, 1997). The use of a wire stylet under ultrasound guidance has been successfully used, either to unblock the inflation channel (Vandermeer and Weatherly, 1989) or to burst the balloon (Carr, 1995). However, one of the most commonly used methods is transrectal, supra-pubic or transperineal puncture (a needle puncture of the balloon, under ultrasound- guided conditions). This has been shown to be a safe and effective method of dealing with balloon non-deflation (Ali Khan *et al*, 1991; Rice and Mogel, 1991).

Fractures

Finally, one other problem has been reported in the literature, although it is not a commonly encountered problem, that of the 'fractured Foley' catheter. A case has been described of a catheter that snapped in half while in place (Harland *et al*, 1992), although the reasons for this are speculative. It has been suggested that it may have resulted from trauma to the catheter within the urethra, some other mechanical defect, or possibly because the catheter had been in place for a long period (over three months). This case serves to provide nurses with a timely reminder to change long-term catheters within the bounds of manufacturers' recommendations so as not to breach their product liability.

Conclusion

Patients with long-term urinary catheters need to be studied from their own unique perspectives (Wilde, 1997). The treatment of catheter problems and the use of solutions must be undertaken only after careful assessment and documentation of the patient and his/her catheter history.

As the breaking of the closed system may introduce infection, this must be considered against the blockage problems of the catheter. The patient's diet and fluid intake is vital in the assessment and the patient should be encouraged to increase oral fluids if possible in order to flush out the catheter him/herself. Decreasing the incidence of catheter blockage by using planned care and individual regimes should lead to less crisis management and more anticipated needs. This is less traumatic for the patient and less demanding on the resources of nursing time and emergency referrals.

It is better to prevent catheter problems, than deal with them as they occur; hopefully, this chapter has provided some useful suggestions that may help if problems do arise.

Key points

❖ Compiling a documented catheter history helps to anticipate and manage blockage problems.

❖ Do not treat bypassing by replacing the catheter with a larger one. Investigate the cause.

❖ Always choose the smallest catheter that will drain adequately.

❖ Always screen for latex allergy before catheterisation is undertaken.

❖ If a catheter is 'rejected' try to find an alternative method of managing urinary problems.

❖ Try simple methods of dealing with balloon non-deflation before resorting to percutaneous puncture.

References

Addison R (1997) *Looking after your Bladder Programme. General Fluid Advice*. Mayday Healthcare, London

Alderman C, ed (1989) Catheter care: nursing standard special supplement. *Nurs Standard* 4(3): supplement

Ali Khan S, Landes F, Paola AS, Ferrarotto L (1991) Emergency management of the non-deflating Foley catheter balloon. *Am J Emerg Med* 9: 260–3

Anders K (1999) Bladder retaining. *Prof Nurse* 14(5): 334–6

Belfield PW (1985) Catheter rejection. *Nurs Times* 81(46 supplement): 67–8

Britton P, Wright ES (1990) Nursing care of catheterized patients. *Prof Nurse* 5(4): 231–4

Bush S (2000) Fluids, fibre and constipation. *Nurs Times Plus* 96(31): 11–12

Carr L (1995) An alternative to managing the non-deflating Foley catheter in women. *J Urol* 153: 716–17

Chrisp JM, Nacey JN (1990) Foley catheter balloon puncture and the risk of free fragment formation. *Br J Urol* 66: 500–2

Cravens D, Zweig S (2000) Urinary catheter management. *Am Fam Physician* 61(2): 369–76

Crow R, Chapman R, Roe B, Wilson J (1986) *A Study of Patients with an Indwelling Urinary Catheter and Related Nursing Practice*. Nursing Practice Research Unit, Guildford

Evans A, Painter D, Feneley R (2001) Blocked urinary catheters: nurses' preventive role. *Nurs Times* 97(1): 37–8

Getliffe KA, Dolman M (1997) *Promoting Continence: A Clinical and Research Resource*. Baillière Tindall, London

Getliffe KA (1996) Bladder instillations and bladder washouts in the management of catheterized patients. *J Adv Nurs* 23: 548–54

Getliffe KA, Hughes SC, Le Claire M (2000) The dissolution of urinary catheter encrustation. *Br J Urology* 85: 60–4

Godfrey H, Evans A (2000) Management of long-term urethral catheters: minimizing complications. *Br J Nurs* 9(2): 74–81

Godwin RJ, Lloyd SN (1990) The non-deflating Foley catheter. *Br J Clin Practice* 44(11): 438–40

Harland RW, DeGroot DL, Dewire D (1992) The fractured Foley: an unusual complication of chronic indwelling urinary catheterization. *J Am Geriatr Soc* 40(8): 827–8

Hedelin H, Bratt CG, Eckerdal G, Lincoln K (1991) Relationship between urease producing bacteria, urinary pH and encrustation on indwelling urinary catheters. *Br J Urol* 67(5): 527–31

Kennedy AP, Brocklehurst JC, Lye MDW (1983) Factors related to problems of long-term catheterization. *J Adv Nurs* 8: 207–12

King JB, Stickler DJ (1992) The effects of repeated instillations of antiseptics on catheter associated urinary tract infections. *Urol Res* 20: 403–7

Kohler-Ockmore J, Feneley RC (1996) Long-term catheterization of the bladder: prevalence and morbidity. *Br J Urol* **77**(3): 347–51

Lowthian P (1995) An investigation of the uncurling forces of indwelling catheters. *Br J Nurs* **4**(6): 328–34

Lowthian P (1998) The dangers of long-term catheter drainage. *Br J Nurs* **7**(7): 366–79

Morris NS, Stickler DJ, Winters C (1997) Which indwelling urethal catheters resist encrustation by Proteus mirabilis biofilms. *Br J Urol* **80**: 58–63

Nazarko L (1998) Back to the future. *Nurs Times* **94**(42 supplement): 79–80, 83–4

Norberg B, Norberg A, Parkhede U (1983) The spontaneous variation in catheter life in long-stay geriatric patients with indwelling catheters. *Gerontology* **29**: 332–5

Norton C (1996) *Nursing for Continence*. Beaconsfield Publishers, Beaconsfield

Read NW, Celik AF, Katsinelos P (1995) Constipation and incontinence in the elderly. *J Clin Gastroenterol* **20**(1): 61–70

Rew M (1999) Use of catheter maintenance solutions for long-term catheters. *Br J Nurs* **8**(11): 708–15

Rice MM, Mogel G (1991) Removal of obstructed Foley catheter from the urethra. *Am J Emerg Med* **9**: 72–3

Rigby D (1998) Long-term catheter care. *Prof Nurse* (Study Supplement) **13**(5): S14–S15

Roe B, Brocklehurst JC (1987) Study of patients with indwelling catheters. *J Adv Nurs* **12**(6): 713–18

Vandermeer JL, Weatherly K (1989) Nursing management of the underflatable Foley catheter balloon. *Home Healthcare Nurse* **8**(5): 39–44

Wilde MH (1997) Long-term indwelling urinary catheter care: conceptualizing the research base. *J Adv Nurs* **25**: 1252–61

Wilson J (1997) Control and prevention of infection in catheter care. *Community Nurse* (Nurse Prescriber) **3**(5): 39–40

Winder A (1994) Suprapubic catheterisation. *Community Outlook* **4**(12): 25–6

Winn C (1998) Complications with urinary catheters. *Prof Nurse* (Study Supplement) **13**(5): S7–10, S16–17

Woodward S (1997) Complications of allergies to latex urinary catheters. *Br J Nurs* **6**(14): 786–93

10

Use of catheter maintenance solutions for long-term catheters

Margaret Rew

This chapter identifies the problems most commonly encountered in the care of patients with long-term indwelling urinary catheters. Using individualised regimens for catheter maintenance solutions (or 'bladder washouts' as they are commonly known) minimises the risk of infection and catheter blockage, thus reducing the need to re-catheterise more than is necessary. Ever since catheters have been used for long-term urinary drainage, problems such as blockage and leakage because of encrustation have caused discomfort to the patient. Another major problem associated with catheter use is the risk of developing a urinary tract infection. Research has shown that with careful management, such as urine testing using a pH indicator strip and use of appropriate solutions, complications can be minimised. Information for this chapter has been obtained via a literature review, interviews and visits with district and hospital nurses, as well as from personal experience.

Catheters have been used for centuries. The term 'catheter' was used by the Greeks in the time of Hippocrates to describe 'an instrument to drain fluid from a body cavity'. The early urinary catheterisations were performed with reeds, straws or tubes of gold or bronze. Different materials have been used over the years and are still being constantly evaluated, reviewed and improved upon today. Dr Frederick Foley designed the catheter in 1930 that now bears his name. The design has not changed since.

Urinary incontinence may be caused by various factors, and the use of long-term catheters as a means of managing incontinence should only be considered as a last resort. Long-term catheters are used most commonly in the elderly and in patients with debilitating neurological conditions. It is with these two groups of patients that most problems occur.

There is a clear correlation between the number of times the drainage system is disconnected and the rate of infection (Getliffe and Dolman, 1997). It is important, therefore, to keep the drainage system closed as much as possible. According to Britton and Wright (1990), the drainage bag should only be disconnected from the catheter:

- when the bag requires changing
- when the catheter becomes blocked
- if catheter maintenance solutions are required.

Based on information already published, observation of current clinical practice and discussion with nurses in hospital and the community, it seems that many nurses indiscriminately perform 'wash-outs' without any clinical reasoning or thought about the effects. It is with this in mind that this literature review has been conducted. It examines the use of 'washouts' (the instillation of fluid into the bladder via a catheter by using a pre-packed solution or in some cases a bladder syringe to either mechanically flush away debris or dissolve developing encrustation) and proposes a more systematic plan of care than is currently in use. A plan of care should involve the factors listed in *Table 10.1*. If necessary,

Table 10.1: Plan of care
A thorough assessment of each patient, eg. diet, mobility, fluid intake and medical history
A review of care at each visit
Regular testing of the urinary pH, eg. weekly or more frequently if the patient is prone to blocking every few days
Building of a catheter history, ie. the length of the catheter life before blocking, cause of blockage, etc
Source: Getliffe (1996)

an appropriate maintenance solution can be used. By adopting this method, the indiscriminate use and abuse of catheter maintenance solutions should be reduced.

Nursing is constantly changing, with new research, developments and attitudes to practice emerging. Nurses are responsible for their own professional practice and educational development. The UKCC recognises that practice must rapidly respond to change and development, so nurses must develop to meet patients' needs. As practitioners, it is essential that we maintain and improve our standards of care. The UKCC's *Code of Professional Conduct* (UKCC, 1992) reminds us to:

- act always in such a way as to promote and safeguard the well-being and interests of the patient/client
- ensure that no action or omission on our part or within our sphere of influence is detrimental to the condition or safety of patients/clients
- take every reasonable opportunity to maintain and improve professional knowledge and competence.

Literature review

Catheter-associated urinary tract infections account for a large number of hospital-acquired infections. Forty-four per cent of hospitalised patients with catheters have been found to develop significant bacteriuria within 72 hours of catheterisation (Crow *et al*, 1986). Some of these infections result in complications including pyelonephritis, epididymitis, abscess formation and chronic renal failure (Warren *et al*, 1987). This leads to increased morbidity and mortality. Catheter blockage, which may lead to such conditions as mentioned above, represents one of the most common complications associated with infections (Elves and Feneley, 1997).

Attempts have been made to improve the methods for the prevention, control and treatment of catheter-associated infections (*Table 10.2*). Once an in-dwelling device, catheter or prosthesis becomes infected, the associated micro-organisms show remarkable resistance to both host defences and antimicrobial agents (Elves and Feneley, 1997). Therefore, although all of these procedures have been shown to either reduce the incidence or delay the onset of catheter-associated infection, they have been unable to eradicate it.

Table 10.2: Methods for the prevention, control and treatment of catheter-associated infections
Avoidance of unnecessary catheterisations
The use of a closed drainage system
Strict observation of aseptic technique in the handling of catheters
The use of cranberry juice drinks
The production of catheters containing antimicrobial substances

Another commonly used method to combat infections and related blockage complications is irrigation of the urinary catheter with various solutions. However, the application of numerous agents using a variety of irrigation methods has resulted in a confusing picture, both in terms of their efficiency and clinical applications.

This review evaluates catheter maintenance solutions for the control of catheter-associated problems and proposes changes to standard irrigation procedures. As previously stated, patients with long-term indwelling urinary catheters are likely to develop a urinary tract infection, and approximately 50% of catheterised patients are susceptible to recurrent catheter encrustation (Getliffe, 1994).

Unchecked encrustation may lead to:

- blockage of the catheter lumen
- bypassing or retention of urine
- pain
- unnecessary catheter changes.

These problems cause distress to the patients and their carers and place increased demands on health service time and resources.

The building up of encrustation and urease activity results in an increase in urine alkalinity (*Figure 10.1*). It has been shown in a study examining the pH and encrustation that patients with a mean urinary pH below 6.8 had minute traces of encrustation, while patients above pH 6.8 had considerably more (Hedelin *et al*, 1991).

Bacteriuria is an inevitable consequence of long-term catheterisation (King and Stickler, 1992), and the source of the infecting organisms is frequently the patient's own bowel. Encrustation occurs on all types of catheter material currently in use; however, different materials have shown to differ in the rate at which they become coated in encrustation. The all-silicone catheters, for example, have been shown to take longer to become encrusted than the silicone-coated, Teflon and latex catheters (Kunin *et al*, 1987).

Hydrogel-coated catheters have shown less susceptibility to encrustation (Talja *et al*, 1990). However, controversy still exists in this area. One study indicated that hydrogel-coated catheters were just as prone to encrustation by *Proteus mirabilis* (one of the most common urease-producing bacteria) as all other types of material used (Morris *et al*, 1997).

The management of catheter encrustation has largely depended on the use of catheter maintenance solutions, or bladder washouts, to relieve blockage. There is, however, little literature examining the efficacy of such solutions in clinical situations. The majority of studies carried out have been under laboratory conditions using a physical model of the catheterised bladder, where different solutions and their effects could be carefully examined. Bach (1990) demonstrated how regular citric acid irrigation reduces crystal deposits on catheters. Further studies have been undertaken linking urinary pH to encrustation.

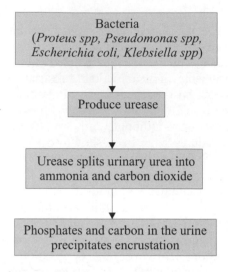

Figure 10.1: Building up of encrustation

The results of one study examining the effectiveness of bladder washouts in reducing catheter encrustation demonstrated that as urinary pH increased, the urine became more opaque and crystallisation was visible on the catheter balloon and drainage tubing (Getliffe, 1994). Furthermore, the effect of using a Suby G or mandelic acid 'washout' solution visibly reduced the opacity of the urine during the time the 'washout' was retained within the catheter and bladder. The mean patent luminal area of the catheter following the use of these solutions was significantly greater than that for controls, which had no solution instilled. Saline solutions did not significantly reduce encrustation compared with controls which had no 'washouts'. The use of saline would be purely mechanical to shift debris. This study demonstrated that both Suby G and mandelic acid were effective in reducing catheter encrustation, but saline had no effect.

Solution R, being double the strength of Suby G, has been used successfully following lithotripsy to dissolve fragments of struvite (a mineral that, along with others, forms the crystals of encrustation and composition of renal calculi) (Holden and Rao, 1991). In the dissolution of catheter encrustation, the use of Solution R may be limited in frequency because of the possibility of producing inflammatory tissue reactions from the stronger acidic solution. However, it may be useful in dissolving encrustations blocking the catheter by instilling it as far as the blockage and leaving it in place for 10–30 minutes (Getliffe, 1996). Solution R may also be instilled before catheter removal. This dissolves external encrustations that cause pain and tissue trauma on withdrawal of the catheter.

Mandelic acid has also been shown to reduce the colony count of several species of micro-organisms forming biofilms on silicone surfaces, including

Escherichia coli, Pseudomonas and *Proteus mirabilis* (Stickler and Hewitt, 1991). Although King and Stickler (1992) have shown that mandelic acid is effective against other organisms, *Proteus mirabilis* is extremely difficult to eradicate from the catheterised bladder. To gain from using mandelic acid, it needs to be used in the very early stages of infection, before the organisms have established themselves in the bladder and colonised on the available surfaces with biofilm.

Chlorhexidine solutions have been used for long-term catheterised patients quite liberally in the past. However, studies have shown that their continuous prophylactic use does not prevent or eliminate the common infecting organisms (King and Stickler, 1992), and may lead to the development and selection of resistant organisms.

The potential risks to the bladder associated with the use of 'washout' solutions have raised concerns. Elliot *et al* (1989) demonstrated an increase in the shedding of urothelial cells following the use of various solutions. The study showed differences in urothelial shedding pre- and post- 'washout'. There was little difference in post-washout shedding depending on the solution used. The response of an increase in shedding cells was suggestive of the physical force of the procedure rather than the chemical irritation.

A catheter lumen holds little more than 4ml and therefore volumes of 50ml or less of catheter maintenance solution will completely fill the catheter lumen and bathe the tip without allowing a large excess of solution to be in contact with the bladder mucosa (Getliffe and Dolman, 1997).

The traditional manner in which 'washouts' have been performed is using a 50–60ml syringe attached to the catheter. The plunger is alternately depressed and withdrawn to facilitate drainage and removal of debris. This may be potentially damaging to the tissues because of the considerable force exerted on the syringe (Getliffe and Dolman, 1997).

Unless indicated, the use of catheter maintenance solutions should be avoided because of the risk of introducing further infection each time the closed system is disrupted. However, for patients whose catheter persistently blocks, the nurse must maintain patient comfort by reducing the need for unnecessary catheter changes, and increasing catheter life. This results in less trauma for the patient and may be cost-effective because of reduced catheter changes (Flack, 1993).

Maintenance solutions

Following a literature review, it is possible to examine practice with regard to the management of patients with indwelling catheters and to recommend changes in the use of catheter maintenance solutions.

Suby G, Solution R and saline solutions are currently available in pre-packed 50ml and 100ml sterile delivery systems. Chlorhexidine and mandelic acid solutions are available in sterile 100ml bags. The solution is warmed to body temperature and the bag is connected to the catheter using an aseptic technique. The contents are emptied into the bladder using the force of gravity. In some instances a gentle squeeze may be required to start the solution flowing into the catheter or if the urine in the catheter is thick with debris.

Catheter maintenance solutions are:

- mandelic acid — 1%
- citric acid — 3.23% (suby g)
- citric acid — 6% (solution r)
- chlorhexidine — 1:5000
- sodium chloride — 0.9% (saline).

Recommendations

The use of all solutions is a matter for professional assessment of the needs of the individual patient. If the patient is newly catheterised, it is wise to monitor how long the first catheter remains *in situ* before showing signs of blockage without the interference of prophylactic 'washouts'. All aspects of catheter care need to be assessed, including: patient activity and mobility; diet and fluid intake; standards of patient hygiene; and the carer's ability to care for the catheter.

A catheter history will be developed and recorded, upon which to base future care regimens and, if indicated, the appropriate use of a 'washout'. For example, to build a clear pattern of catheter history, it has been suggested that between three and five consecutive catheters should be observed (Norberg *et al*, 1983). It is then possible to diagnose the cause of any blockage problems.

The use of pH indicator papers is advisable to help assess the alkalinity of the urine and, if monitored regularly, eg. weekly or more frequently, if the blockages occur very frequently. Collection of a urine sample for micro-biological analysis may be indicated to isolate any specific infecting organisms that require systemic antibiotics.

If encrustation is identified a citric acid washout regimen may be commenced and increased or decreased as necessary. The encrustation is identified by removing the blocked catheter, observing the tip upon which crystals of encrustation may adhere, and splitting the catheter along its length to observe if encrustation has adhered to the lumen of the catheter.

If blockage problems are caused by debris, such as shedding urothelial cells, mucus or small blood clots, a saline 'washout' may be indicated.

By careful monitoring of the catheter history and accurate documentation of the treatment given, the patient's catheter problems may be more easily managed. The solutions may be given between twice daily or once a week depending on the severity of the problem. It is recommended that mandelic acid be used for a maximum of three weeks if a patient has an infection such as Pseudomonas (Robertson and Norton, 1990).

Conclusion

It has been shown that it is possible to reduce massive crystal deposits on the catheter by regular irrigation of the catheter with citric acid solutions (Bach, 1990). Decreasing the incidence of catheter blockage by using individual regimens with effective solutions can increase the catheter life. This is less traumatic for the patient and may be more cost-effective than recatheterisation (Flack, 1993).

Even with modern drainage systems, nearly all the patients undergoing catheterisation develop a urinary tract infection. Infections with urease-producing micro-organisms — even when asymptomatic — produce an alkaline urine. This provides the ideal conditions for the formation of crystals. Crystal deposits act as a niche for infecting organisms, rendering it refractory to treatment. A vicious cycle of infection/crystallisation occurs. The availability of the various catheter maintenance solutions provides the flexibility to break this cycle. By careful monitoring, a maintenance regimen that suits the individual patient and keeps the catheter patent may be established.

Key points

❖ When undertaking catheter care management it is vital to thoroughly assess the patient's diet, fluid intake and lifestyle.

❖ An accurate catheter history must be documented upon which to base care regimes and assess results.

❖ It is important to choose the correct solution once the cause of the blockage has been established.

❖ Nurses can monitor the success of the regime by observing the length of time the catheter takes to block and by testing the pH of urine for alkalinity.

❖ Each patient is an individual case and must therefore have his/her own plan or regime of care specific to his/her catheter management.

References

Bach D (1990) Prophylaxis against encrustation and urinary tract infection with in-dwelling transurethral catheters. *Urolog Nephrol* **2**(1): 25–32

Britton PM, Wright ES (1990) Nursing care of catheterised patients. *Profess Nurse* **5**(5): 231 4

Crow R, Chapman R, Roe B, Wilson J (1986) *A Study of Patients with an In-dwelling Urinary Catheter and Related Nursing Practice.* Nursing Practice Research Unit, Guildford

Elliot TSJ, Reid L, Gopal Rao G, Rigb RC, Woodhouse K (1989) Bladder irrigation or irritation *Br J Urol* **64**: 391–4

Elves AWS, Feneley RCL (1997) Long-term urethral catheterisation and the urine biomate *J Urol* **80**:1–5

Flack S (1993) Finding the best solution. *Nurs Times* **11**: 68–74

Getliffe KA (1994) The use of bladder washouts to reduce urinary catheter encrustation. *Br J Urol* **73**: 696–700

Getliffe KA (1996) Bladder installations and bladder washouts in the management of catheterised patients. *J Adv Nurs* **23**: 548–54

Getliffe KA, Dolman M (1997) *Promoting Continence: A Clinical and Research Resource.* Baillière-Tindall, London

Hedelin H, Iratt CG, Eckerdal G, Lincoln K (1991) Relationship between urease producing bacteria, urinary pH and encrustation on in-dwelling urinary catheters. *Br J Urol* **67**(5): 527–31

Holden D, Rao PN (1991) Management of staghorn stones using a combination of lithotripsy, percutaneous nephrolithotomy and Solution R irrigation. *Br J Urol* **67**: 13–7

King JB, Stickler DJ (1992) The effects of repeated installations of antiseptics on catheter-associated urinary tract infections. *Urological Res* **20**: 403–7

Kunin CM, Chin QF, Charnbers S (1987) Formation of encrustation on in-dwelling urinary catheters in the elderly. *J Urol* **77**(3): 347–51

Morris NS, Stickler DJ, Winters C (1997) Which in-dwelling urethral catheters resist encrustation by *Proteus mirabilis* biofilms. *Br J Urol* **80**: 58–63

Norberg B, Norberg A, Parkhede U (1983) The spontaneous variation in catheter life in long-stay geriatric patients with in-dwelling catheters. *Gerontology* **29**: 332–5

Robertson DJ, Norton MS (1990) The effect of 1% mandelic acid as a bladder irrigation fluid in patients with in-dwelling catheters. *Br J Clin Practice* **44**(8): 142–4

Stickler DJ, Hewitt P (1991) Activity of antiseptics against biofilms of mixed bacterial species growing on silicone surfaces. *Eur J Clin Microbiological Infection* **10**: 416–21

Talja M, Korpela A, Jarvi K (1990) Comparison of urethral reaction to full silicone hydrogel coated and siliconised latex catheters. *Br J Urol* **66**: 652–7

Warren JW, Damorn D, Tonney JH, Hoopes JM, Deforege B, Munrie HL (1987) Fever, bacteruria and death as a complication of bacteruria in women with long-term urethral catheters. *J Infectious Diseases* **155**: 1151–8

UKCC (1992) *Code of Professional Conduct for the Nurse, Midwife and Health Visitor.* UKCC, London

11

Bladder washouts in the management of long-term catheters

Ann Evans and Helen Godfrey

It has been estimated that 40–50% of patients with long-term catheters can suffer with catheter blockage. This not only causes distress to the patient but also increases the demands on community nurses' time and resources. Infection with bacteria such as *Proteus* causes the urine to become alkaline. Crystalline deposits can then form inside the catheter lumen which causes blockage. Nurses often manage blocked catheters with the use of bladder 'washouts' or bladder instillations. However, the literature is confused over the terminology of 'bladder washouts', instillations and irrigation and a great deal of controversy surrounds the effectiveness of these procedures. Crisis management of catheters occurs when nurses wait for catheters to become blocked before changing them; this often occurs at inconvenient times and patients frequently have to wait several hours before help is available. To avoid crisis management, nurses should aim to assess individual patients' 'pattern of catheter life' and plan changes accordingly. This would improve patient care and allow nurses to utilise their time more effectively.

Approximately 4% of patients cared for by district nurses in the community have indwelling urinary catheters (Roe, 1989; Getliffe, 1990). One recurring aspect of their management concerns the use of 'bladder washouts' to prolong catheter life. Within the nursing literature the subject is confused not only by different terminology relating to 'bladder washouts', 'bladder irrigation' and 'bladder instillations', but also by the effectiveness of these procedures in reducing encrustation.

Recently, the term 'catheter maintenance solutions' has been introduced, and this seems to be a more generic term which embraces the different types of solutions and approaches (Rew, 1999). Patients with long-term catheters will almost inevitably have bacteriuria and urinary tract infections are prevalent (Willis, 1995; Wilson, 1998). Associated complications are catheter encrustation and subsequent blockage although some patients have minimal complications.

This chapter will explore two main issues in catheter management. First, it will attempt to clarify the terminology and, second, examine the available evidence for performing these procedures in the clinical setting.

Catheter blockage

The morbidity and burden of long-term catheterisation to the patient, carer, nurse and healthcare manager are substantial. Sassoon *et al* (1991) demonstrated that 43% of long-term catheterised patients experience problems and over 50% suffer with catheter blockage (Getliffe, 1990). This often leads to crisis management of catheters with the catheter being changed when it becomes acutely blocked rather than the catheter change being planned (Getliffe, 1994a).

Catheter blockage can be very distressing for patients and places extra demands on nursing time and resources (Getliffe, 1990). Frequently, catheter blockage cannot be managed in the community because many trusts require staff to have undertaken further training before they can perform male and suprapubic catheterisation. Since there is an insufficient number of staff in the community trained in these skills, patients with blocked catheters tend to rely on the accident and emergency departments to have their catheters changed (Kohler-Ockmore, 1992).

Catheter blockage occurs when urine is unable to flow through the catheter; it is often caused by a build up of deposits within the catheter lumen. Bacteriuria is inevitable for patients with indwelling long-term catheters (Crow *et al*, 1986). Bacteria such as *Proteus* in the urine cause alkalinity which is associated with encrustation (Wiseman, 1997).

The main cause of encrustation is mineral deposits of struvite (aluminium magnesium phosphate) and apatite (calcium phosphate) (Getliffe, 1996). Normal urine pH is less than 7, but the formation of struvite occurs when the urine pH is 7.2 (Getliffe and Mulhull, 1991). Morris *et al* (1997) undertook tests on all available catheters and found that none of them were resistant to encrustation. However, the all-silicone catheters took less time to block and it was suggested that this could be due to the larger lumen size of this type of device.

Washouts, irrigation or instillations?

Getliffe (1994b) argues that the management of blocked catheters depends mainly on the use of 'bladder washouts'. The term 'bladder washout' appears to be a generalised term for introducing and withdrawing fluid into the bladder. Bladder instillations and bladder irrigation are frequently referred to as 'bladder washouts'.

This implies that there is some confusion in the terminology, which could have significant implications in practice and the appropriate choice of procedure. To minimise confusion the three procedures have been distinguished and classified (*Table 11.1*).

Despite the controversy surrounding the use of bladder instillations and washouts, a recent study shows they are still widely used. Forty-two per cent of individuals with suprapubic catheters received some form of bladder maintenance solution within the last year (Evans and Feneley, 2000). Instillations commonly used for managing catheter-associated complications included Suby G and Solution R

(Evans and Feneley, 2000). These commonly used bladder maintenance solutions (eg. Uro-Tainer, B/Braun Medical Ltd, Aylesbury) are attributed by the manufacturer to have the features outlined in *Table 11.2*.

Table 11.1: Definitions of bladder irrigation, washouts and instillations	
Bladder irrigation	Continuous bladder irrigation is the means by which sterile fluid (usually saline) is used to irrigate the bladder using a three-way catheter, irrigation giving-set and a catheter drainage bag. This is used after urological surgery to prevent clot retention (Gilbert and Gobbi, 1989)
Bladder washouts	Traditionally, bladder washouts have been performed to actively flush the bladder and disturb debris, or to reduce or prevent catheter obstruction. This is achieved using a 60ml bladder syringe with saline and alternately depressing and withdrawing the plunger until the debris is removed (Kennedy, 1984)
Bladder Instillations	Bladder instillations can be described as the use of a prepacked sterile reagent (usually 100ml) which is allowed to flow into the bladder under gravity by raising the bag of instillation fluid above the height of the bladder. The fluid is retained in the bladder (usually about 15 minutes) and then allowed to drain out under gravity (Getliffe, 1996)

Table 11.2: Bladder maintenance solutions	
Suby G	Citric acid (3.23%), used to dissolve or reduce crystallisation in the bladder or catheter
Solution R	Citric acid (6%), used to dissolve persistent crystallisation or to minimise trauma on catheter removal
Chlorhexidine	Chlorhexidine (0.02%) used to reduce bacterial growth
Mandelic acid	Mandelic acid (1%), used to reduce the growth of urease-producing bacteria, *Proteus* and *Pseudomonas*
It is recommended that all of these solutions be used twice daily or weekly depending on the severity of the case	

Getliffe (1994b) states that there has been much controversy concerning the use of bladder washouts and instillations, as it is believed that their use can damage the bladder mucosa either as a result of the reagent or the physical forces used. Elliot *et al* (1989) suggest that the bladder mucosa has an important role against fighting infection in the bladder. In many published articles, instillations and irrigation are referred to as 'washouts'; therefore, it is hardly surprising that nurses are confused by the terminology.

Use of irrigation, washouts and instillations

Getliffe (1994a) used synthetic urine in a bladder model system to show the effects of Suby G, mandelic acid and saline to reduce catheter encrustation. These results identified that Suby G and mandelic acid were effective in reducing encrustation, but saline was not. This chapter discusses the use of 'bladder washouts'; however, the procedure described was an instillation. This again highlights the need to define terminology.

Kennedy (1984) studied the effects of Suby G on 15 patients and found that it significantly reduced catheter encrustation compared to saline. Kennedy *et al* (1992) conducted a randomised cross-over study of three bladder instillations — Suby G, Solution R and saline in 25 female patients with indwelling long-term catheters. These findings suggest that saline is ineffective at reducing encrustations.

However, in this study the authors discuss the use of both bladder washouts and instillations, but do not specify the procedures associated with the different terminology, again adding to the confusion. Although struvite crystals were present in the returned acidic instillations it was felt that there was no significant difference in catheter encrustation between the various instillations. This suggests that instillation of weak acidic solutions did not effectively reduce catheter encrustation.

During this study it was noted that there was a high percentage of red blood cells in the fluid drained from the bladder following Suby G treatment, suggesting that acidic solutions may damage the bladder endothelium. Also, this study demonstrated that all the returned 'washout' fluid from the patients contained high levels of urothelial cells. Elliot *et al* (1989) suggested that bladder irrigation can lead to an increased shedding of urothelial cells, but the actual method described in this study is a slow instillation — again confusing. Getliffe (1996) indicates that instillations may reduce the risks of damage to the bladder, because there is no force used to instil the reagent. However, research suggests that despite the minimal forces used during instillations, the bladder mucosa can still be damaged and predispose patients to urinary tract infection (Kennedy *et al*, 1992).

Stickler *et al* (1987) showed that chlorhexidine bladder washouts were ineffective in preventing infection caused by the use of long-term catheters. However, Getliffe (1994a) identified that chlorhexidine 'bladder washouts' were still being used by 47% of nurses who performed washouts. Getliffe (1994a) discusses the use of washouts but it is unclear as to whether the solutions were administered as a 'washout' or as an 'instillation'.

Getliffe (1994a) identified that the percentage of patients receiving bladder washouts had fallen to 36%. Previous work by Getliffe (1990) showed that 54% of nurses used bladder washouts; Roe (1990) identified that this figure was 44%. However, in this article it is unclear which was used — washout or instillation. Fewer bladder washouts were done because research suggested they might have a detrimental effect on the bladder (Elliot *et al*, 1989; Kennedy *et al*, 1992). As mentioned earlier, a recent study investigating current nursing management of long-term suprapubic catheters found that 42% of patients received bladder instillations (Evans and Feneley, 2000).

Roe (1989) argued that there was a lack of sound scientific knowledge about the use of bladder washouts. This is reiterated in the literature which suggests that the evidence surrounding the use of 'washouts' remains confusing and conflicting (Kohler-Ockmore, 1991; Getliffe 1996).

The current management of blocked catheters depends largely on the use of washouts/instillations or frequent catheter changes (Getliffe, 1996). To avoid damaging the mucosa, Getliffe (1996) suggests that a much smaller amount of acidic solution could be used which just fills the catheter. Therefore, it is hoped that the catheter encrustation would be reduced with minimal damage to the bladder, but clinical research would be needed to ascertain if such practice is effective.

A recent *in vitro* study using a catheterised bladder model suggests that smaller volumes of Suby G (50ml) were as effective as 100ml used in practice and two sequential washouts (50ml) are more effective than a single washout (Getliffe *et al*, 2000).

Kunin *et al* (1987) indicate that patients with long-term catheters can be divided into two groups — those that regularly block (blockers), and those whose catheters do not block (non-blockers). Patients whose catheters frequently block may benefit from having their catheters changed every 7–10 days (Kunin *et al*, 1987). By carefully monitoring patients with long-term catheters it is possible to establish a 'characteristic pattern of catheter life' (Norberg *et al*, 1983; Getliffe, 1996). If catheter life can be predicted then nurses may be able to change the catheter before it blocks, thus avoiding 'crisis management' of catheters. Bladder instillations seem to be an expensive way of prolonging catheter life with possible detrimental effects to the patient (Getliffe, 1996).

Conclusion

This chapter has described how confusing the terminology is surrounding the use of bladder irrigation, washouts and instillations and that they are all different ways of administering solutions into the bladder.

For future practice it may cause less confusion if the methods of administrating a solution into the bladder were more accurately used:

- a bladder irrigation is the administration of fluid (usually saline) via a three-way catheter and irrigation set into the bladder following urological surgery to prevent clot retention
- a bladder washout is the administration of a solution (usually saline) manually into the bladder to remove debris, using a bladder syringe, alternately depressing and withdrawing the plunger until the debris is removed
- a bladder instillation is a prepacked sterile reagent (usually 100ml) that is allowed to drain into the bladder under gravity. The fluid is retained in the bladder for a specified time (usually 15 min) and then allowed to drain out under gravity.

In vitro studies indicate that weak acidic solutions are effective in reducing catheter encrustation; however, the clinical studies undertaken are inconclusive. The literature also reveals that washouts and instillations may have detrimental effects on the bladder.

The literature on the use of bladder washouts and instillations remains confusing and conflicting. Over the last ten years there have been several articles written on the use of bladder washouts but their efficacy is unproven.

It is necessary to break the closed drainage system when solutions are used as bladder washouts, instillations and irrigations. Getliffe (1997) argues that breaks in the closed drainage system should be as infrequent as possible to minimise bacterial access into the catheter.

The literature suggests that it may be possible to predict the life of a catheter by monitoring urine pH levels, and change the catheter when the individual patient's blocking pH has been reached. Clinical research is needed to assess the effectiveness of such catheter management.

To avoid crises with catheters it seems reasonable that nurses should try to predict individual patients' catheter life pattern and aim to change the catheter before it blocks. Regular testing of the urine pH may predict the catheter life and this suggests that more clinical research needs to be done.

Key points

❖ There is confusion in the nursing literature over the terms 'bladder washouts', 'bladder irrigation' and 'bladder instillations'.

❖ Controversy surrounds the use of catheter maintenance solutions in the management of blocked catheters.

❖ Nurses should aim to be proactive in the management of long-term catheter care.

❖ Nurses should change catheters before they block in patients who have this tendency.

References

Crow R, Chapman R, Roe B, Wilson J (1986) *Study of Patients with an Indwelling Urethral Catheter and Related Nursing Practice.* Nursing Practice Research Unit, University of Surrey, Guildford

Elliot P, Reid L, Gopol Rao G, Rigby R, Woodhouse K (1989) Bladder irrigation or irritation. *Br J Urol* **64**: 391–4

Evans A, Feneley R (2000) A study of current nursing management of long-term suprapubic catheters. *Br J Comm Nurs* **5**(5): 240–5

Getliffe K (1990) Catheter blockage in community patients. *Nurs Standard* **5**(9): 33–6

Getliffe K (1994a) The characteristics and management of patients with recurrent blockage of long- term urinary catheters. *J Adv Nurs* **20**: 140–9

Getliffe K (1994b) The use of bladder washouts to reduce urinary catheter encrustation. *Br J Urol* **73**: 696–700

Getliffe K (1996) Bladder instillations and bladder washouts in the management of catheterised patients. *J Adv Nurs* **23**: 548–54

Getliffe K (1997) Catheters and catheterisation. In: Getliffe K, Dolmon M, eds. *Promoting Continence: A Clinical and Research Resource*. Baillière Tindall, London: 281–341

Getliffe K, Hughes S, Le Claire M (2000) The dissolution of urinary catheter encrustation. *Br J Urol* **85**: 60–4

Getliffe K, Mulhull A (1991) The encrustation of indwelling catheters. *Br J Urol* **67**: 337–41

Gilbert V, Gobbi M (1989) Making sense of bladder irrigation. *Nurs Times* **85**(16): 40–2

Kennedy A (1984) Trial of a new bladder washout system. *Nurs Times* **80**(46): 48–51

Kennedy A, Brocklehurst J, Robinson J, Faragher E (1992) Assessment and the use of bladder washouts/instillations in patients with long-term indwelling catheters. *Br J Urol* **70**: 610–5

Kohler-Ockmore J (1991) Chronic urinary catheter blockage. *Nurs Standard* **5**(44): 26–8

Kohler-Ockmore J (1992) Urinary catheter complications. *J District Nurs* **10**(8): 18–20

Kunin C, Quee Fah Chin B, Chambers M (1987) Indwelling urinary catheters in the elderly. *Am J Med* **82**: 405–11

Morris N, Stickler D, Winters C (1997) Which indwelling catheters resist encrustation by *Proteus mirabilis* biofilms? *Br J Urol* **80**: 58–83

Norberg B, Norberg A, Parkhede U (1983) The spontaneous variation of catheter life in long-stay geriatric inpatients with indwelling catheters. *Gerontology* **29**: 332–5

Rew M (1999) Use of catheter maintenance solutions for long-term catheters. *Br J Nurs* **8**(11): 708–15

Roe B (1989) Use of bladder washouts: a study of nurses' recommendations. *J Adv Nurs* **14**: 494–500

Roe B (1990) Nursing practice for catheter care. *Nurs Practice* **3**(3): 6–9

Stickler D, Clayton C, Chawla J (1987) Assessment of antiseptic bladder washout procedures using a physical model of the catheterised bladder. *Br J Urol* **60**: 413–18

Sassoon E, Abercrombie F, Goodrum P (1991) The permanent indwelling catheter: a domiciliary survey. *Health Trends* **23**(3): 109–11

Willis J (1995) Catheters: urinary tract infections. *Nurs Times* **91**(35): 48–9

Wilson J (1998) Control and prevention of infection in catheter care. *Nurse Prescriber/Community Nurse* **3**(5): 48–9

Wiseman O (1997) Management of the long-term urinary catheter in the asymptomatic patient in the accident and emergency department. *Br J Urol* **80**: 748–51

12

Management of long-term urethral catheters: minimising complications

Helen Godfrey and Ann Evans

Urinary tract infections, tissue damage and encrustation of the catheter, which may cause blockage, are all complications that can arise during long-term catheterisation. It is important for nurses to provide effective catheter care in order to minimise the incidence of these complications. There is still controversy in the nursing literature about certain aspects of catheter management. This chapter explores a number of aspects of catheter care and suggests a rationale for effective and safe management, including the choice of catheter, choice of drainage system, care of the individual and the care of catheter and drainage system.

Long-term catheters are best avoided as they are associated with many complications such as urinary tract infections (UTIs), tissue damage, encrustation of the catheter and blockage (Lowthian, 1998). Long-term catheterisation should only be used as a last resort in the management of urinary incontinence and patients need to be assessed carefully before a urinary catheter is inserted (Rew, 1999). The objectives of effective catheter care are to prevent or minimise the complications related to catheterisation, to promote the independence, comfort and dignity of the patient and to ensure that patients and their carers are knowledgeable and proficient in the management of long-term catheters (Getliffe, 1996; Woollons, 1996; Winson, 1997). The service provided should also be cost-effective (Getliffe, 1996; Woollons, 1996).

It has been suggested that nurses lack the necessary knowledge to provide optimum care for patients with long-term catheters (Crumney, 1989; Henry, 1992; Winn, 1996; Woollons, 1996). Since an indwelling catheter is the main factor which predisposes individuals to UTIs (Mulhall, 1991), it is important for nurses to provide effective catheter care to minimise the incidence of UTIs and the complications that can result. UTIs associated with long-term catheters result from bacteria gaining entry to the bladder via two possible routes: the catheter lumen or the space between the walls of the catheter and the urethra (Gould, 1994; Willis, 1995). Other complications which can arise during long-term catheterisation are tissue damage and encrustation of the catheter which may cause blockage.

Many authors have set out the principles of catheter care (Gould, 1994; Getliffe, 1996; Pomfret, 1996; Parker, 1999); however, there is still much controversy and debate about certain aspects of catheter care resulting in confusion about how best to approach the management of long-term catheters.

This chapter will principally examine how the incidence and complications of UTIs associated with long-term catheterisation can be minimised. In addition, it will address aspects of catheter management which seek to minimise tissue trauma and problems of catheter encrustation which is linked to UTI (Morris *et al*, 1997; Rew, 1999). Key aspects of catheter management are highlighted in *Table 12.1*.

A number of aspects of catheter management will be discussed in the chapter; these include: care of the individual; choice of catheter; choice of drainage system; and care of catheter and drainage system.

Catheter length and size

The length of catheter can influence the incidence of infection since kinks forming in the tubing can prevent effective drainage. Prevention of kinks in the tubing is part of effective infection control practice (Wilson, 1997). Therefore, a catheter of appropriate length should be selected as excess catheter can result in loss of dignity and increase risk of trauma or blockage due to kinking. Woollons (1996) suggests that a suitable catheter length is 41–42cm for males and 25cm for females. Getliffe (1996) suggests a 45cm catheter length for males and 25cm for females.

There is apparent consensus in the literature regarding the optimum size of catheter which should be selected. Catheter size is usually measured in Charrière (Ch) units which refer to the outer circumference of the catheter. This is approximately three times the external diameter of the catheter, thus a 12Ch catheter has an external diameter of 4mm.

The principle is to choose the smallest diameter catheter that allows for effective drainage which is commonly 12–14Ch (Woollons, 1996). Getliffe (1996) recommends a catheter size of 12–16Ch which reflects the sizes proposed by Gould (1994) of 12–16Ch for men, and 12–14Ch for women.

Larger size catheters can cause pain and discomfort (Roe and Brocklehurst, 1987). It is also suggested that larger catheters cause irritation, trauma and the bypassing of urine and may increase the risk of infection (Pomfret, 1996). Larger catheters are also associated with abscess formation (Roe and Brocklehurst, 1987). However, catheters with a larger diameter may be required if clots are present in the urine.

Catheter material

The relationship between catheter material, bacterial infection and encrustation is widely acknowledged and some materials are preferred for long-term use. There are a wide range of catheter materials available and the material selected should be chosen for the following characteristics: comfort; ease of insertion and removal; and ability to reduce the likelihood of complications such as tissue damage, colonisation by micro-organisms and encrustation (Getliffe, 1996; Woollons, 1996).

Table 12.1. Key aspects of catheter management

Action or characteristic	Rationale	References
Care of the individual		
Maintain a high fluid intake	To prevent dehydration and constipation For adequate flushing of bladder and to produce dilute urine. This may also limit the likelihood of catheter encrustation and catheter-associated infection	Pinkerman (1994), Wilson (1997), Roe (1993), Getliffe (1997)
Wash hands before and after emptying catheter bag	To reduce the risk of cross infection	Gould (1994), Getliffe (1996)
Use new gloves when emptying catheter bag	To reduce the risk of cross infection	Gould (1994), Getliffe (1996), Winson (1997)
Wash perianal and meatal areas using soap and water	To remove urethral secretions which if left may form hard crusts and cause trauma when catheter is removed To reduce risk of infection	Burke *et al* (1983), Falkiner (1993), Willis (1995), Getliffe (1996), Winson (1997)
Choice of catheter		
Optimum catheter length for individual (45cm males, 25cm females)	To prevent kinks forming To maintain discreteness and enhance aesthetic appearance	Getliffe (1996), Woollons (1996), Winson (1997), Lowthian (1998)
Smallest size of catheter which will allow free drainage of urine (usually 12–14Ch)	To prevent irritation, trauma and pain To prevent passing of urine To reduce incidence of infection	Getliffe (1996), Woollons (1996), Winson (1997), Parker (1999)
Choose all silicone or hydrogel-coated catheters for long-term catheterisation	To minimise incidence of encrustation and subsequent blockage	Lowthian (1998), Winn (1998)
Change catheters proactively in individuals prone to catheter blockage	To avoid catheter becoming blocked and preventing crisis management	Getliffe (1994), Getliffe (1997), Wiseman (1997)
Change catheters according to manufacturer's recommendations for individuals who are not prone to catheter blockage	To minimise the number of occasions in which the closed drainage system is broken To avoid discomfort of unnecessary catheter change	Woollons (1996), Lowthian (1998)
Choice of drainage system		
Select bag with an appropriate volume	To ensure bag is fit-for-purpose, ie. will accommodate sufficient urine in order that it does not have to be emptied too frequently	Getliffe (1996), Winson (1997)
Choose suitable tap and non-return valve	To ensure the tap can be easily opened and closed To prevent backflow of urine	Getliffe (1997
Presence of self-sealing sample port	To minimise the risk of infection when taking a urine sample	Gould (1994)
Maintenance of drainage system		
Maintain closed system	To minimise risk of infection	Pinkerman (1994), Wilson (1997)
Change bags at intervals of 5–7 days	To reduce the risk of infection by breaking closed system	Department of Health (1992)
Bag should be supported adequately and positioned below the bladder	To prevent the backflow of urine To prevent discomfort and dragging on the catheter	Getliffe (1996), Wilson (1997), Lowthian (1998)
Empty catheter bag into clean container	To reduce the risk of cross infection	Gould (1994), Getliffe (1996), Parker (1999)
Wash hands and wear new gloves each time the catheter bag is emptied	To reduce the risk of infection and cross infection	Wilson (1997), Winson (1997), Parker (1999)
Avoid using bladder washouts and instillations	To reduce the risk of infection To prevent trauma to bladder mucosa	Pinkerman (1994), Wilson (1997), Wiseman (1997), Rew (1999)
Avoid using antibiotics in the treatment of asymptomatic bacteriuria	To minimise the risk of antibiotic resistant bacteria emerging	Getliffe (1996), Wiseman (1997), Rew (1999)

All-silicone catheters and hydrogel-coated catheters are less likely to encrust (Winn, 1998). It is suggested that all-silicone Foley catheters with smooth-edged drainage eyes are the optimum choice for long-term catheterisation (Curran, 1992; Lowthian, 1998). However, the balloon in all-silicone catheters allows some diffusion of water and on occasion may deflate *in situ* (Getliffe, 1996). In a study of the encrustation of different catheter materials using a model catheterised bladder (Morris *et al*, 1997), all catheters blocked but the all-silicone catheters took longer to block than other types. However, this may be because all-silicone catheters have a slightly wider lumen than other coated catheters (Morris *et al*, 1997).

Catheter balloon size

While the balloon is critical for retention of the catheter *in situ* its size should be chosen to minimise risks of irritation, spasm and mechanical damage. Woollons (1996) suggests that a balloon with a capacity for 5–10ml of water should be selected. Getliffe (1996) recommends a balloon capacity of 10ml. The balloon should be filled according to the manufacturer's instructions since underfilling or overfilling may interfere with the correct positioning of the catheter tip which may lead to irritation and trauma of the bladder wall (Woollons, 1996; Getliffe, 1997).

Larger balloon catheters should not be selected to reduce the risk of expulsion as balloon sizes of 30ml can press on the bladder or urethral tissue causing ulceration and possible stricture formation (Getliffe, 1997; Parker, 1999).

Frequency of catheter change

According to the nursing literature, the frequency of catheter change is variable. Woollons (1996) suggests that catheters should remain in place for the maximum manufacturer's recommended time as replacement increases the risk of infection and is an unpleasant experience. Lowthian (1998), however, recommends that catheters are changed every five days or even twice a week, arguing that frequent catheter changes minimise the hazards associated with abrasion due to encrustation on the catheter tip and balloon surface.

Some individuals experience catheter blockage due to encrustation within a few days while others have catheters *in situ* for weeks to months without forming encrustations (Kunin, 1989). This suggests that catheters should be changed proactively according to the individual's usual pattern of catheter life rather than being replaced after they become blocked (Getliffe, 1994, 1997).

Drainage system

A wide range of drainage bags are available and individuals should be able to choose from a selection of bags with an appropriate volume, suitable tap and non-return valve (Getliffe, 1996; Winson, 1997). In addition, a self-sealing sample port should be present in order that urine samples can be removed without breaking the closed system (Gould, 1994). The principle is to promote independence and self-care by enabling individuals to choose drainage systems which suit their needs. This includes ensuring that the type of bag is comfortable to wear and that the tap can be easily opened and closed (Getliffe, 1997).

For some individuals a catheter valve may be more appropriate than a drainage system as it enables the individual to empty his/her bladder intermittently. The type of valve chosen must match the individual's ability to manipulate it (Getliffe, 1997).

Position of bag

The position of the bag is critical and must ensure good drainage and prevent backflow of urine. The drainage bag should be placed below the level of the bladder (Getliffe, 1996), but should not be more than 30cm below it as the negative pressure created may cause the bladder mucosa to be sucked into the 'eyes' of the catheter (Lowthian, 1998).

Drainage bag support

As the drainage bag fills with urine it becomes heavy and could drag uncomfortably if not suitably supported. There are different ways of supporting the drainage bag including the use of a stand, a hanger attached to the bedframe or a device to support the drainage bag on the body. Body-worn bags are available with a variety of supporting mechanisms including a holster suspended from the waist or a sporran (Getliffe, 1997). Smaller leg bags which are strapped to the leg or held in place with a net sleeve or stocking can be used during the daytime and these can be secured to the thigh or calf (Getliffe, 1996).

Bag change

When the closed system is broken micro-organisms may be introduced to the drainage system, thus disconnection of the catheter from the catheter bag should be avoided. Since changing the bag is associated with cross infection (Platt *et al*, 1983) it is recommended that the drainage bag is changed at intervals of 5–7 days (Department of Health, 1992). Others suggest that the drainage bag is renewed each time the catheter is changed (Lowthian, 1998). Some argue that there is no evidence to suggest that drainage bags need to be changed at specific intervals, but should only be changed when they are blocked by deposits or are damaged (Wilson, 1997).

Hygiene

When emptying the catheter bag it is important to recognise that the urine is likely to be contaminated with large numbers of micro-organisms. The risks of cross infection can be significantly reduced if hands are washed and new gloves are worn when a catheter bag is emptied. Patients at home should wash their hands before and after emptying their catheter bags. Nurses should avoid emptying catheter bags from a number of patients in turn using one container and one pair of gloves. Containers used to collect urine should be thoroughly cleaned and dried between use (Gould, 1994; Getliffe, 1996). In relation to personal hygiene, washing the perianal and meatal areas daily with soap and water to remove urethral secretions is adequate (Willis, 1995; Getliffe, 1996; Winson, 1997) since the use of antiseptics does not appear to prevent infection or abolish existing infection (Burke *et al*, 1983; Falkiner, 1993; Parker, 1999).

Diet

Maintaining a high fluid intake is thought to produce a less concentrated urine which impairs bacterial growth in the drainage bag. In addition, the flushing action of larger quantities of dilute urine will reduce the likelihood of bacteria ascending from the bag (Wilson, 1997) and flush micro-organisms out of the bladder (Roe, 1993).

In addition, dilute urine may reduce the concentration of substances leading to precipitation and encrustation. Getliffe (1997) suggests that while there is no evidence to indicate that drinking large amounts will reduce the incidence of catheter encrustation or catheter-associated infections, a sufficient fluid intake will prevent constipation and dehydration.

Cranberry juice is increasingly being employed to prevent and treat UTIs (Nazarko, 1995; Leaver, 1996). However, some suggest it is uncertain whether a high intake of cranberry juice or ascorbic acid to achieve a lower urinary pH has a beneficial effect on increasing catheter life or reducing infection rates (Roe, 1993; Getliffe, 1996). One study, a randomised, double-blind, placebo-controlled trial, demonstrated that cranberry juice has a more significant effect in clearing infected urine of bacteria rather than in preventing the occurrence of UTI (Avorn *et al*, 1994).

It is considered that cranberry juice has several therapeutic properties including the prevention of bacterial adherence to mucosa (Leaver, 1996). Since adherence to mucosa is necessary before infection can occur (Pinkerman, 1994), this may be the basis of the therapeutic action of cranberry juice.

Bladder instillations and washouts

Of all aspects of catheter care, bladder instillations and washouts are the most controversial (Pomfret, 1996). In the past, bladder washouts and instillations were employed to minimise the likelihood of catheter-associated UTIs and to dissolve encrustations or clear blockages. The evidence to support this aspect of catheter care practice is absent from the literature although instillations are still widely used (Roe, 1993; Pinkerman, 1994). Wilson (1997) argues that bladder instillations are a potential hazard because they increase the risk of introducing micro-organisms as their administration involves breaking the closed drainage system.

Wiseman (1997) suggests that the optimum management of a blocked catheter should be to change the catheter rather than performing a bladder washout in an attempt to clear the blockage.

Conclusion

The guiding principle for effective catheter management always involves addressing the individual needs of the patient (Willis, 1995; Woollons, 1996). The aim of effective catheter care is to minimise the incidence of complications which include UTIs, tissue damage and encrustation of the catheter which may lead to catheter blockage.

Key points

- ❖ A major complication of long-term catheterisation is the development of urinary tract infections.

- ❖ Effective catheter management aims to prevent or minimise the complications related to long-term catheterisation.

- ❖ Nurses should base their care of the individual with a long-term catheter on a clear rationale.

- ❖ The individual needs of the patient should be addressed in all aspects of catheter care.

References

Avorn J, Monane M, Gyrwitz JH, Glynn RJ, Choodnovsky I, Lipsitz LA (1994) Reduction of bacteriuria and pyruria after ingestion of cranberry juice. *J Am Med Assoc* **271**(10): 751–4
Burke JP, Jacobson JA, Garibaldi RA, Conti MT, Alling DW (1983) Evaluation of meatal care with polyantibiotic ointment in prevention of urinary catheter associated bacteriuria. *J Urology* **120**: 331–4
Crumney V (1989) Ignorance can hurt. *Nurs Times* **85**(21): 65–70

Curran E (1992) A programme to audit the use of urinary catheters. *J Clin Nurs* **1**: 329–34

Department of Health (1992) *Drug Tariff*. HMSO, London

Falkiner FR (1993) The insertion and management of indwelling urinary catheters — minimising the risk of infection. *J Hosp Infec* **25**: 79–90

Getliffe K (1994) The characteristics and management of patients with recurrent blockage of long-term urinary catheters. *J Adv Nurs* **20**: 1140–9

Getliffe K (1996) Care of urinary catheters. *Nurs Standard* **11**(11): 57–60

Getliffe K (1997) Catheters and catheterisation. In: Getliffe K, Dolman M, eds. *Promoting Continence: A Clinical and Research Resource*. Ballière Tindall, London: 281–341

Gould D (1994) Keeping on tract. *Nurs Times* **90**(40): 58–63

Henry M (1992) Catheter confusion. *Nurs Times* **88**(42): 65–72

Kunin CM (1989) Blockage of urinary catheters: role of micro-organisms and constituents of the urine on formation of encrustations. *J Clin Epidemiol* **42**(9): 835–42

Leaver R (1996) Cranberry juice. *Prof Nurse* **11**(8): 525 6

Lowthian P (1998) The dangers of long-term catheter drainage. *Br J Nurs* **7**(7): 366–79

Morris NS, Stickler DJ, Winters C (1997) Which indwelling urethral catheters resist encrustation by *Proteus mirabilis* biofilms? *Br J Urol* **80**: 58–63

Mulhall AB (1991) Biofilms and urethral catheter infections. *Nurs Standard* **5**(18): 26–8

Nazarko L (1995) The therapeutic uses of cranberry juice. *Nurs Standard* **9**(34): 33–5

Parker LJ (1999) Urinary catheter management: minimising the risk of infection. *Br J Nurs* **8**(9): 563–74

Pinkerman ML (1994) Indwelling urinary catheters. *Nurs* **94**: 66–8

Platt R, Polk BF, Murdock B, Rosner B (1983) Reduction of mortality associated with nosocomial urinary tract infection. *Lancet* **i**: 893–7

Pomfret IJ (1996) Catheters: design, selection and management. *Br J Nurs* **5**(4): 245–51

Rew M (1999) Use of catheter maintenance solutions for long-term catheters. *Br J Nurs* **8**(11): 708–15

Roe BH (1993) Catheter-associated urinary tract infection: a review. *J Clin Nurs* **2**: 197–203

Roe BH, Brocklehurst JC (1987) Study of patients with indwelling catheters. *J Adv Nurs* **12**: 713–18

Willis J (1995) Catheters: urinary tract infections. *Nurs Times* **91**(35): 48–9

Wilson J (1997) Control and prevention of infection in catheter care. *Nurse Prescriber/Community Nurse* **3**(5): 39–40

Winn C (1996) Catheterisation: extending the scope of practice. *Nurs Standard* **10**(52): 49–54

Winn C (1998) Complications with urinary catheters. *Prof Nurs* **13**(Supplement 5): S7–S10

Winson L (1997) Catheterisation: a need for improved patient management. *Br J Nurs* **6**(21): 1229–32

Wiseman O (1997) Management of the long-term urinary catheter in the asymptomatic patient in the accident and emergency department. *Br J Urol* **80**: 740 51

Woollons I (1996) Urinary catheters for long-term use. *Prof Nurse* **11**(12): 825–32

13

Complications of allergies to latex urinary catheters

Sue Woodward

Latex products are widely used both in our homes and in hospitals. Latex allergy is an increasingly worrying problem for health professionals, not least allergy to latex urinary catheters. The pathophysiology of latex allergy is discussed with reference to catheter allergy. Other known problems of latex catheters are also highlighted, including toxicity leading to urethritis and stricture formation, and encrustation. Nurses need to be aware of the increasing incidence of latex allergy and the importance of screening patients specifically for this risk factor.

Urinary catheters have been used throughout the ages. The first were simple metal tubes used for the treatment of urinary retention from the third century BC (Bloom *et al*, 1994). These tubes were rigid, either straight or slightly curved, with a hole at the tip and often had a blunted end. The insertion of rigid catheters was known to cause trauma and attempts were made to overcome this problem by the use of more malleable instruments, usually made from silver (Nacey and Delahunt, 1993).

Eventually, flexible catheters were designed; these were fashioned from a metal spiral covered with a soft material such as parchment covered with wax. More durable, flexible catheters became possible after 1844, when vulcanisation of rubber was perfected (Marino *et al*, 1993). Flexible catheters made entirely of rubber replaced the metal ones and became widely used by the end of the nineteenth century. The resulting catheter was relatively durable, flexible and easily introduced, and marked the beginning of the modern catheter used today (Nacey and Delahunt, 1993). In the early 1900s, many new plastic materials became available and these were soon used in the production of urinary catheters. These materials, eg. Silicone, Teflon coatings and polyvinylchloride (PVC), caused less urethritis and encrustation than latex catheters; however, many clinicians still preferred the latex versions. There is now a preference for silicone or coated latex catheters, which tend to be non-toxic because of their coating (Nacey and Delahunt, 1993); however, coating a latex catheter does not appear to afford protection against latex allergy as will be discussed later.

No catheters available before the early nineteenth century were able to be retained in the bladder. It was not until then that balloons, fashioned from animal gut, were secured to the tip of the catheter, allowing them to be held in place. In the 1930s, Frederick Foley utilised rubber balloon catheters and championed the manufacture of the balloon and catheter in one piece by their serial agglutination of layers of latex on a metal form. Current balloon catheters are made predominantly by bonding a separate balloon onto the surface of a catheter.

This chapter focuses on some of the modern complications of catheterisation with latex urinary catheters, namely latex allergy and encrustation. This will be illustrated by the case of Mrs A.

Case history

Mrs A was a 45-year-old lady who had been admitted to a regional neurosurgical unit for removal of a recurrent meningioma. Post-operatively Mrs A developed urinary retention and was catheterised with a polytetra-fluoroethylene (PTFE)-coated (previously known as Teflon-coated) latex catheter, size 12Ch with a 10ml balloon filled with sterile water. Three days after catheter insertion Mrs A was noticed to have a redness over her vulval area and a white exudate. She was assumed to have vaginal *Candida albicans* infection and was treated with a clotrimazole pessary; however, the situation did not improve. Two weeks following catheterisation the catheter began bypassing and Mrs A was recatheterised using a Bard Biocath (hydrogel) 12Ch female length catheter. This remained *in situ* for a further week and the bypassing continued, as did the redness and exudate.

At this point Mrs A's husband remembered that she had previously developed a contact dermatitis to latex condoms. Once it was realised that Mrs A's problem could be due to the latex catheters, she was recatheterised using a 100% silicone catheter. Within days the bypassing had stopped and the redness and exudate caused by the contact dermatitis rapidly resolved.

Pathophysiology of latex allergy

The frequency of hypersensitisation to latex has been increasing (Chamboyron *et al*, 1992) since it was first documented by Nutter in 1979. The prevalence of contact dermatitis to rubber is also on the increase (Bayrou, 1993). Latex (natural rubber) is a highly processed plant product derived from the sap of the rubber tree Hevea brasiliensis. It contains proteins, lipids, amino acids, nucleotides, cofactors and abundant cis 1,4 polyisoprene. It is this last product that is purified and vulcanised using heat and sulphur to make rubber (Slater, 1989). Allergic reactions to latex are classified into two main types: type I (antibody-mediated) immediate and type IV (cell-mediated) delayed response (Barton, 1993).

Latex is mainly composed of large molecules and has not been shown to cause type IV allergies itself, but the vulcanisers and chemicals used in the manufacturing process are frequently responsible for sensitisation (Conde-Salazar *et al*, 1993). These are readily liberated in a warm, humid environment, such as a patient's urethra. The prevalence of type IV reactions is approximately 3.8–7.35% (Bayrou, 1993) and symptoms are exhibited within 24–48 hours of contact (Pecquet, 1993).

Patients with a type I hypersensitivity appear to have an immunoglobulin E(IgE)-mediated reaction to *H. brasiliensis* proteins that persist in the final product (Kerner and Newman, 1993). The symptoms associated with each type of allergy are summarised in *Table 13.1* (Barton, 1993).

It is known that certain individuals are more susceptible to latex allergy and that allergic reactions usually occur after repeated exposure to products made from or containing latex. Healthcare workers are particularly at risk owing to frequent contact with latex gloves, as are people involved in the manufacture of latex products (Kerner and Newman, 1993). Also at risk are patients with an atopic history (history of asthma, hay fever, rhinitis, or eczema), and those who have undergone multiple surgical procedures and suffered frequent exposure to latex gloves and healthcare products (Barton, 1993).

There are many reports in the literature of allergy to latex household items such as rubber gloves, and any patient with a history of rubber allergy should be treated with caution. There is a need to identify patients at risk as those who have previously had a mild reaction may develop an anaphylactic response on further exposure (Kerner and Newman, 1993). *Table 13.2* summarises the most common items to which allergy to latex has been reported.

Table 13.1: Type I reactions and type IV contact dermatitis reactions.	
Type I reactions	Local urticaria
	Systemic urticaria
	Rhinitis
	Asthma
	Conjunctivitis
	Shock
	Bronchospasm
	Anaphylaxis
Type IV reactions	Erythema
	Pruritus
	Scaling
	Vesicles
	Papules

Table 13.2: Items which are known to cause a type I or type IV latex allergy in sensitised individuals	
Condoms	Rademaker and Forsyth, 1989; Lezaun *et al*, 1992; Bircher *et al*, 1993
Balloons (especially children)	Kerner and Newman, 1993
Household rubber gloves	Belsito, 1990
Wheelchair tyres	Belsito, 1990
Underwear elastic	Conde-Salazar, 1990
Eyelash curlers	Vestey *et al*, 1985
Garden hose and electrical vibrator	Effendy *et al*, 1992

Latex allergy has also been associated with medical products manufactured from latex, most commonly surgical gloves (Conde-Salazar, 1990; Smart and Lawrence, 1992; Mansell *et al*, 1994), but also red rubber ventricular shunts (Woodruff *et al*, 1986), dental dams (Smart and Lawrence, 1992), enema catheters (Sissons and Evans, 1991), and urinary catheters (Axelssonn *et al*, 1988; Gonzalez, 1992; Barton, 1993).

In clinical practice, however, many cases of rubber allergy are not adequately diagnosed (Ancona *et al*, 1990) or are simply overlooked (Rademaker and Forsyth, 1989; Bircher *et al*, 1993). Many health professionals do not recognise patients at risk, as was the case with Mrs A, and a simple screening question as to whether she had ever experienced any adverse reactions to rubber products would have prevented a great deal of discomfort. In this case, also, the type IV allergic reaction was not recognised and it is possible that many other patients are inappropriately treated because their allergy to latex urinary catheter goes undiagnosed.

Patients at risk of latex allergy need to be identified. Nurses are in an ideal position to undertake this screening by asking a few simple questions to identify risk factors, as highlighted previously. Perhaps every patient should be screened for latex allergy before catheterisation with a latex catheter. Patients with a known or suspected allergy to latex require teaching regarding their condition and protection from future reactions.

Toxicity of latex catheters

Latex catheters have also been implicated in the development of urethritis and urethral strictures, a subject on which there has been much debate. In 1982, an epidemic of urethral stricture following catheterisation with latex catheters was reported by Ruutu *et al*. Urethritis is a common complication of urethral catheterisation and may result in stricture formation (Nacey *et al*, 1985). This was shown by Ruutu *et al* (1982) in cardiac surgery patients who underwent urinary catheterisation. The authors subsequently changed their practice and used silicone catheters, with no incidence of stricture formation thereafter (Ruutu *et al*, 1984). The uncoated latex catheters used were subsequently found to contain substances that were toxic to cells *in vitro* (Graham *et al*, 1983). Before 1982, there had been little regulation of the standards of catheter manufacture or acceptable levels of toxicity. Standards were then produced for catheter toxicity, and in the UK cytotoxicity tests for medical rubber and plastics were developed and published as BS 5736 (Robertson, 1992).

In order to comply with the new standards, a range of coated catheters was produced: silicone or PTFE was used to coat the latex. A hydrogel-coated catheter is now also available (Nacey and Delahunt, 1991). The hydrogel-coated catheter has been the subject of much research since its introduction, and *in vitro* studies have demonstrated that it will reduce the high level of cytotoxicity associated with latex catheters to a level akin to that associated with pure silicone catheters (Nacey and Delahunt, 1991). Many coatings provide an unreliable barrier to the diffusion of toxic products from the underlying latex, whereas the hydrogel coating remains largely intact during use (Cox, 1987). This may explain why hydrogel catheters cause less urethritis and stricture formation. However, the hydrogel coating does not appear to provide protection against an allergic reaction to the underlying latex, as demonstrated by the case of Mrs A. This may be because hydrogel coatings have poor insulating properties against water-soluble chemicals dissolving from the latex core (Talja *et al*, 1990). Silicone catheters should therefore still be used in these cases.

Catheter material and encrustation

Another problem associated with long-term urinary catheterisation is encrustation. This is formed from mineral salts that precipitate from the urine onto the catheter. Encrustation occurs in up to 50% of patients with long-term catheters *in situ*. This again is a particular problem with the use of latex catheters (Talja *et al*, 1990; Bach *et al*, 1990; Bull *et al*, 1991) and is reduced with the use of silicone catheters (Binder and Gonick, 1969; Talja *et al*, 1990). Surface coatings have been designed to resist encrustation.

It has been suggested that increased encrustation is associated with the higher rate of urethritis that is seen with latex catheters. If this is the case, then a silicone catheter may protect an individual from the problems of encrustation because it causes less urethritis (Nacey *et al*, 1985). It would then follow that a hydrogel-coated latex catheter which produces a similar incidence of urethritis to that associated with silicone catheters should also present less problems with encrustation.

Hydrogel is an inert and highly biocompatible substance. It coats the catheter inside and out and has been given a zero toxicity rating by the British Standards criteria (Bull *et al*, 1991). These authors conducted a study to assess the degree of encrustation on hydrogel-coated catheters when compared with catheters coated with other materials. It was found that the hydrogel-coated catheters were preferred by patients, were able to remain *in situ* for longer and were associated with reduced rates of bypassing (often a sign of encrustation or urethral inflammation). The results obtained by Bull *et al* (1991) confirmed the findings of *in vitro* studies undertaken by Cox (1987), who reported that a hydrogel-coated latex catheter minimises encrustation. Cox (1987) found specifically that the Bard Biocath (a hydrogel catheter) resisted encrustation as well as, but no better than, 100% silicone catheters.

The Biocath produces less friction on insertion and removal (Nickel *et al*, 1987) and this surface smoothness may be a factor in reducing bacterial cell adhesion to the catheter (biofilm) and subsequent encrustation (Cox, 1987). Bacterial colonisation has been implicated in encrustation formation. As bacteria build up within the bladder, the urinary pH changes from acidic to alkaline. The alkaline environment allows the deposition of mineral salts on the catheter. It has now been shown that use of an acidic bladder washout (Suby-G or Mandelic Acid Urotainer) will significantly reduce the degree of encrustation on a catheter (Getliffe, 1994a) and can resolve the problem of catheter blockage in an acute situation.

Conclusion

For many patients the problems associated with latex catheters, namely allergy, toxicity and encrustation, are distressing and the cause of significant morbidity. They also increase the demands upon nursing time and resources, with patients often requiring re-catheterisation, when this may have been avoidable. Nurses are ideally placed to prevent the development of these problems through screening patients for allergy before catheterisation, for example, and the selection of a catheter manufactured from appropriate material. If nurses are aware of the signs and symptoms of latex allergy or toxicity, they can detect such problems at an earlier stage and act upon them. Encrustation can be prevented by the use of a prophylactic regimen of urotainer bladder washouts and selection of an appropriate catheter material for the individual patient. For some patients it may be possible to identify a pattern of catheter blockage (Getliffe, 1994b) and, having achieved this, proactively undertake a programme of planned recatheterisation rather than reacting to an acutely blocked catheter. If these points are borne in mind, perhaps fewer patients will suffer the same fate as Mrs A, or suffer urethral trauma as a catheter encrusted with crystals is removed via their urethra, causing abrasions.

PTFE-coated latex catheters will continue to be used, as they cost less than hydrogel-coated or silicone catheters. Coated latex catheters also have a lower incidence of balloon deflation, as a result of the process by which they are manufactured, than all-silicone catheters. Nurses will need to be more vigilant and specifically screen and monitor patients for risk of developing latex allergy to urinary catheters.

Key points

* ❖ Urinary catheters made from latex are in common usage.

* ❖ Latex has been shown to cause contact dermatitis and in some cases hypersensitivity and anaphylaxis. These allergic reactions to latex are occurring with increasing frequency.

* ❖ Latex allergy is often missed; nurses should be aware of the possibility and screen patients who may be at risk.

* ❖ Patients who are known to be allergic to latex or are thought to be at risk, and who require urinary catheterisation, should be catheterised using pure silicon urethral catheters.

References

Ancona A, Arevalo A, Macotela E (1990) Contact dermatitis in hospital patients. *Dermatol Clin* **8**(1): 95–105

Axelsson IG, Eriksson M, Wrangsjo K (1988) Anaphylaxis and angioedema due to rubber allergy in children. *Acta Paediatr Scand* **77**: 314–6

Bach D, Hesse A, Prange CH (1990) Prophylaxis against encrustation and urinary tract infection with indwelling transurethral catheters. *Urol Nephrol* **2**(1): 25–32

Barton EC (1993) Latex allergy: recognition and management of a modern problem. *Nurse Pract* **18**(11): 54–8

Bayrou O (1993) Epidemiology of type IV allergies to rubber chemical additives. *Clin Rev Allergy* **11**: 421–5

Belsito DV (1990) Contact urticaria caused by rubber-analysis of seven cases. *Dermatol Clin* **8**(1): 61–6

Binder CA, Gonick P (1969) Experience with silicone rubber-coated foley urethral catheters. *J Urol* **101**: 716–8

Bircher AJ, Hirsbrunner P, Langauer S (1993) Allergic contact dermatitis of the genitals from rubber additives in condoms. *Contact Dermatitis* **28**: 125–6

Bloom DA, McGuire EJ, Lapides J (1994) A brief history of urethral catheterisation. *J Urol* **151**: 317–25

Bull E, Chilton CP, Gould AL, Sutton TM (1991) Single-blind randomised, parallel group study of the Bard Biocath catheter and a silicone elastomer coated catheter. *Br J Urol* **68**: 394–9

Chambeyron C, Dry J, Leynadier F, Pecquet C, Tran Xuan Thao (1992) Study of the allergenic fractions of latex. *Allergy* **47**: 92–7

Conde-Salazar L (1990) Rubber dermatitis: clinical forms. *Dermatol Clin* **8**(1): 49–55

Conde-Salazar L, del-Rio E, Guimaraens D, Domingo AG (1993) Type IV allergy to rubber additives: a 10-year study of 686 cases. *J Am Acad Dermatol* **29**: 176–80

Cox ASJ (1987) Effect of a hydrogel coating on the surface topography of latex-based urinary catheters: an SEM study. *Biomaterials* **8**: 500–1

Effendy I, Geiler U, Bischoff R, Happle R (1992) Anaphylaxis due to a latex vaginal vibrator. *Contact Dermatitis* **27**: 318–9

Getliffe KA (1994a) The use of bladder wash-outs to reduce urinary catheter encrustation. *Br J Urol* **73**: 696–700

Getliffe KA (1994b) The characteristics and management of patients with recurrent blockage of long-term urinary catheters. *J Adv Nurs* **20**: 140–9

Gonzalez E (1992) Latex hypersensitivity: a new and unexpected problem. *Hosp Pract* **27**: 32–51

Graham DT, Mark GE, Pomeroy AR (1983) Cellular toxicity of urinary catheters. *Med J Austr* **1**: 456–9

Kerner MM, Newman A (1993) Diagnosis and management of latex allergy in surgical patients. *Am J Otolaryngol* **14**(6): 440–3

Lezaun A, Marcos C, Martin JA, Quirce S, Gomez MLD (1992) Contact dermatitis from natural latex. *Contact Dermatitis* **27**: 334–5

Mansell PI, Reckless JPD, Lovell CR (1994) Severe anaphylactic reaction to latex rubber surgical gloves. *Br Med J* **308**: 246–7

Marino RA, Mooppan UMM, Kim H (1993) History of urethral catheters and their balloons: drainage, anchorage, dilation and haemostasis. *J Endourol* **7**(2): 89–92

Nacey J, Delahunt B (1991) Toxicity study of first and second generation hydrogel-coated latex urinary catheters. *Br J Urol* **67**: 314–6

Nacey J, Delahunt B (1993) The evolution and development of the urinary catheter. *Aust NZ J Surg* **63**: 815–9

Nacey J, Tulloch AG, Ferguson AF (1985) Catheter-induced urethritis: a comparison between latex and silicone catheters in a prospective clinical trial. *Br J Urol* **57**: 325–8

Nickel JC, Olson ME, Costerton JW (1987) In vivo coefficient of kinetic friction: study of urinary catheter biocompatibility. *Urology* **29**(5): 501–3

Nutter AF (1979) Contact urticaria to rubber. *Br J Dermatol* **101**: 597–8

Pecquet C (1993) Allergic contact dermatitis to rubber. *Clin Rev Allergy* **11**: 413–9

Rademaker M, Forsyth A (1989) Allergic reactions to rubber condoms. *Genitourin Med* **65**: 194–5

Robertson GSM (1992) Letter to the editor. *Br J Urol* **70**: 335–6

Ruutu A, Alfthan O, Heikkinen L, Jarvinen A, Lehtonen T, Merikallio E, Standertskjold-Nordenstam CG (1982) 'Epidemiol' of acute urethral stricture after open-heart surgery. *Lancet* **23**: 218

Ruutu A, Alfthan O, Heikkinen L, Jarinen A, Konttinen M, Lehtonen T, Merikallio E, Standerskjold-Nordenstam CG (1984) Unexpected urethral strictures after short-term catheterisation in open heart surgery. *Scand J Urol Nephrol* **18**: 9–12

Sissons GR, Evans C (1991) Severe urticarial reaction to rubber: complication of a barium enema. *Clin Radiol* **43**(4): 288–9

Slater JE (1989) Rubber anaphylaxis. *N Engl J Med* **320**(17): 1126–30

Smart ER, Lawrence CM (1992) Allergic reactions to rubber gloves in dental patients: reports of three cases. *Br Dent J* **172**: 445–7

Talja M, Korpela A, Jarvi K (1990) Comparison of urethral reaction to full silicone, hydrogel-coated and siliconised latex catheters. *Br J Urol* **66**: 652–7

Vestey JP, Buxton PK, Savin JA (1985) Eyelash curler dermatitis. *Contact dermatitis* **13**(4): 274–5

Woodruff WW, Yea-e AE, Dent GA (1986) Ventricular shunt therapy of the brain: long-term rubber-catheter-induced inflammation. *Radiology* **158**: 171–4

14

Catheterisation and urinary tract infections: microbiology

Helen Godfrey and Ann Evans

Patients with urinary catheters are a substantial proportion of the total patient population and catheter care is an important area of nursing practice. Urinary tract infection associated with catheterisation is known to be the most common nosocomial (hospital-acquired) infection. Urinary tract infections can be caused by exogenous micro-organisms or endogenous faecal or urethral micro-organisms. The different micro-organisms which are responsible for causing urinary tract infections have particular characteristics. Many micro-organisms form a biofilm, a living layer of cells which stick to the surfaces of the catheter and the catheter bag. Biofilms not only lead to urinary tract infections, but also they are associated with encrustation and catheter blockage. The chapter considers the micro-organisms implicated in catheter-associated urinary tract infections and aims to develop an increased awareness of the characteristics of different pathogens which could lead to enhanced nursing practice and improved patient care.

Nurses are responsible for the management of patients with urinary catheters in all settings and specialties. Catheterisation may be necessary for a variety of reasons and once a catheter has been in place for 28 days or more this is considered long-term catheterisation (Winson, 1997). At any given time a significant proportion of patients may have catheters *in situ*. The number of patients with long-term catheters represents 4% of the community workload and 28% of patients cared for in residential homes have long-term indwelling catheters (Getliffe, 1995). About 10% of patients admitted to hospital will have an indwelling catheter inserted (Mulhall *et al*, 1988a,b).

The importance of nurses having the appropriate knowledge and skills to enhance the care of patients with long-term indwelling catheters is further supported by the significant incidence of catheter-associated urinary tract infections (UTIs). An indwelling catheter is the main factor which predisposes patients to UTIs and it is important that nurses have the knowledge to provide optimal care to minimise the problems of UTIs (Mulhall, 1991). This includes delaying the onset of infection in the short-term, preventing cross-infection in catheterised patients and minimising the incidence of complications associated with UTIs.

UTI associated with catheterisation is known to be the most common hospital-acquired infection, possibly accounting for up to 45% of all hospital infections (Winn, 1996). The risk of UTI increases by 5–8% a day of catheterisation (Mulhall *et al*, 1988a,b) and is inevitable in long-term catheterised patients (Getliffe, 1996). Nearly 80% of UTIs are associated with indwelling catheters (Pinkerman, 1994). Catheter-associated UTIs not only make people feel unwell, but also are responsible for mortality (Kunin *et al*, 1992).

UTIs associated with long-term catheterisation represent a significant challenge in nursing practice and an understanding of the microbiology of UTIs can both inform and transform nursing care. There are indications that many nurses appear to lack the knowledge necessary to provide optimal care for a catheterised patient (Crumney, 1989; Henry, 1992; Winn, 1996; Woollons, 1996).

This chapter will give an overview of the microbiology of catheter-related UTIs and will aim to develop an enhanced awareness of the characteristics of different micro-organisms required to support effective nursing care and which could lead to improved nursing practice. The sources and spread of infection will be discussed and the possible complications of urinary tract infections considered.

Bacteriuria or urinary tract infection?

There is a tendency for the terms 'bacteriuria' and 'urinary tract infection' to be used interchangeably in the nursing literature, but while many patients with indwelling catheters have bacteriuria, the presence of bacteria in urine does not imply a diagnosis of UTI (Higgins, 1995). Many patients with bacteriuria do not necessarily show symptoms of infection. Urine is an optimal medium where bacteria can multiply, but even when bacteria are present in the bladder a UTI is not inevitable, provided the bladder is healthy and free from trauma.

Infection usually results from a lowered resistance to disease (Lowthian, 1998). Winson (1997) argues that infection is an inevitable consequence of long-term catheterisation and because chronic bacteriuria can result in bacteraemia or neoplastic changes in the bladder (Stickler and Zimakoff, 1994), encrustation and blockage, then bacteriuria should not be viewed with complacency (Morris *et al*, 1997). Bacteriuria is a common consequence of catheterisation since 44% of hospitalised patients with catheters develop bacteriuria within 72 hours of catheterisation (Crow *et al*, 1986).

The bacteria found in patients with asymptomatic bacteriuria are usually a mixture of the normal bacterial flora of the urogenital tract and perineum. Bacteria will only cause symptomatic infection when tissue invasion occurs. In an attempt to distinguish between bacteriuria and UTI in non-catheterised individuals, some consider that a bacterial count of 10^5 organisms/mm^3 confirms a UTI. However, in some individuals a count of 10^5 organisms/mm^3 does not produce symptoms of infection while in others a lower bacterial count can produce symptoms of UTI (Higgins, 1995).

UTI is associated with signs and symptoms such as pyrexia, pyuria, dysuria, urinary bypassing of the catheter, cloudy foul-smelling urine and, in elderly people, an acute confusional state (Pinkerman, 1994; Getliffe, 1996; Parker, 1999). Signs and symptoms will only occur when the bacteria have invaded the bladder mucosa causing inflammation (Pinkerman, 1994).

Routes of infection

Micro-organisms gain access to the urinary tract through two possible routes, from the catheter lumen or via the space between the walls of the catheter and the urethra, the periurethral route (Willis, 1995; Getliffe, 1996). In addition, since the urethra is colonised by bacteria, the catheter may pick up organisms during insertion which can then be transmitted to the bladder (Pinkerman, 1994).

Biofilms

Since urine is an ideal medium for bacterial growth, bacteria can quickly multiply in the catheter bag. Many micro-organisms form a biofilm, a living layer of cells which stick to the surfaces of the catheter and catheter bag. A biofilm can be described as a collection of micro-organisms and their extracellular products which are bound to a solid surface (Mulhall, 1991). Biofilms have been found on a variety of catheter materials.

Many bacteria can advance up the walls of the drainage bag and other parts of the drainage system against the flow of urine by means of their biofilm (Lowthian, 1998). Bacteria can reach the bladder within a few days (Stickler, 1996) although some suggest biofilms grow slowly (Getliffe, 1996). Incorrect positioning or inadvertent pressure on the drainage bag may facilitate retrograde movement of colonised urine from the bag to the bladder although most bags are fitted with a valve that prevents backflow (Getliffe, 1996).

It is important for nurses to understand the nature of biofilms since not only can biofilms lead to UTIs, but also they are associated with encrustation and blockage, an important complication of long-term catheterisation (Burr and Nuseibeh, 1993; Lowthian, 1998). If the bacteria in the biofilm (eg. *Proteus mirabilis*) produce an enzyme, urease, the biofilm quickly becomes encrusted with struvite or similar mineral deposits (Getliffe and Mulhall, 1991; Morris *et al*, 1997). A catheter can become blocked by an encrusted biofilm within about 24 hours of the biofilm reaching the catheter's lumen (Lowthian, 1998).

The formation of biofilms involves the glycocalyx produced by bacteria. This is a polysaccharide outer layer which helps the bacteria attach to surfaces and to each other forming microcolonies. Most bacteria seem to prefer growing attached to a surface rather than existing free in an aqueous phase. Once bacteria attach and adhere to a surface, the cells surround themselves with glycocalyx and divide by binary fission within the biofilm matrix to form adherent microcolonies. The biofilm matrix may act as a reservoir from which bacteria can detach and cause contamination of the surrounding medium (Khardori and Yassien, 1995).

Biofilms were present in 48.5% of catheters examined in an analysis of 33 indwelling catheters (Ramsay *et al*, 1989). This study also revealed that the bacteria found in the urine were not necessarily the same as those found in the biofilm; this has implications for antibiotic susceptibility testing done on a urine sample, since this may not predict successful antimicrobial activity against the biofilm-associated bacteria (Ramsay *et al*, 1989).

However, it is suggested that antibiotics usually fail to eradicate infection associated with a biofilm, and since micro-organisms are cemented to the surface of the catheter and other parts of the drainage system, the glycocalyx (which they produce) may protect them not only from host-defence mechanisms, but also from the action of antimicrobial agents (Ramsay *et al*, 1989). Other mechanisms of resistance to antimicrobial agents could also be important (Ramirez De Arrellano *et al*, 1994). Use of antibiotics in these circumstances may cause substitution by a more resistant micro-organism (Khardori and Yassien, 1995).

Micro-organisms responsible for urinary tract infections

Bacteria can cause UTIs when they invade the mucosa (Pinkerman, 1994), but there are other characteristics which make bacteria cause disease including: survival on mucosal surfaces, growth in the host's tissue, interference with host defences and damage to the host (Smith, 1995). An appreciation of the different types of bacteria which frequently cause catheter-associated UTIs and their particular characteristics may help nurses provide optimal care and alert them to complications including potential catheter blockage by micro-organisms associated with biofilms, urease production and encrustation.

UTIs can be caused by exogenous micro-organisms such as *Pseudomonas aeruginosa* or by endogenous faecal or urethral micro-organisms (Winson, 1997). The micro-organisms responsible for UTIs are usually the microbial flora found in the gut and are always present as a potential source of reinfection (Getliffe, 1996). The endogenous micro-organisms responsible for UTIs include *Escherichia coli, Staphylococcus epidermidis, S. saprophyticus, Proteus spp.* and *Klebsiella spp.* (Ayliffe *et al*, 1991; Gould, 1994; Higgins, 1995; Winson, 1997).

Table 14.1 shows the most common types of bacteria causing UTIs found in a study of individuals with long-term catheters with the micro-organisms listed in order of prominence (Kohler-Ockmore and Feneley, 1996).

In Kohler-Ockmore and Feneley's (1996) study, 177 urine samples contained mixed cultures while 51 samples were pure cultures. The types of micro-organisms which cause UTIs associated with long-term catheters are different from those involved in UTIs in general (Higgins, 1995). Some suggest that

Table 14.1: The most common types of bacteria causing urinary tract infections in individuals with long-term catheters	
Micro-organism	Coliforms
	Streptococcus faecalis
	Proteus spp.
	Pseudomonas spp.
	Staphylococcus aureus
	Escherichia coli
	Klebsiella spp.
Source: Kohler-Ockmore and Feneley (1996)	

UTIs associated with an indwelling urinary catheter should be viewed as 'complicated urinary tract infections' (Gantz and Noskin, 1997). It is considered that uncomplicated UTIs (those without a urinary catheter) are invariably associated with a single bacterial species, most commonly *E. coli*, but complicated UTIs (with a catheter) are more likely to involve multiple or unusual micro-organisms (Gantz and Noskin, 1997).

Pathogens causing UTIs have different characteristics, eg. *Klebsiella* bacteria are often found in patients who have been treated with antibiotics. *Proteus spp.* causes encrustation because it secretes urease, an enzyme which breaks down urea into ammonium ions. This makes the urine more alkaline and an alkaline urine encourages the precipitation of the insoluble salts calcium and magnesium phosphates (Gould, 1994). *Proteus* bacteria are often associated with the growth of calculi in the kidney and bladder. Certain strains of *Proteus* and *E. coli* have tiny, hair-like processes on their surface, pili, which enable them to adhere to the bladder mucosa (Gould, 1994; Smith, 1995).

Types of *Proteus* which possess pili are more likely to ascend the urinary tract leading to pyelonephritis than strains lacking pili. Certain strains of *S. epidermidis* appear to be successful urinary pathogens because they are able to attach to the surface of catheters (Ramirez De Arrellano *et al*, 1994). The different characteristics of bacteria which are found in catheter-associated UTIs are summarised in *Table 14.2*.

Sources of infection

There is much discussion about the source of pathogens responsible for catheter-associated infection (Gould, 1994). As has been mentioned earlier, the source of infection can be endogenous or exogenous (Winson, 1997). Pathogens are considered to reach the bladder by two possible routes: migration from urine in the catheter bag or via the space between the catheter and urethral mucosa (Gould, 1994; Pinkerman, 1994; Getliffe, 1995).

During the 1960s a closed drainage system was introduced which dramatically reduced the incidence of infection (Roe, 1993; Gould, 1994; Winn, 1996). However, pathogens can gain access to this 'closed system' of drainage in a number of ways, through the drainage tap or at the junction between the catheter and catheter bag, on the catheter tip during insertion, during disconnection and by migration on the inside or outside of the catheter (Pinkerman, 1994).

Kennedy *et al* (1983) identified that patients were more likely to develop bacteriuria if their drainage bags were changed more frequently than patients whose bags remained in place for longer periods. Getliffe (1995) states that to minimise the risks of catheter-associated infection it is necessary to reduce the risks of cross-infection. This can be achieved by maintaining the closed drainage system and engaging in effective hand washing techniques.

The hands of the nurse, patient or carer can be contaminated with a large number of pathogens when handling the drainage bag and the container into which the bag is emptied. The risks of cross-infection can be reduced if hands are thoroughly washed and new gloves are worn each time a catheter bag is emptied.

The container in which the catheter bag is emptied can also be a source of infection. A study by Crow *et al* (1986) showed that nurses frequently used unclean containers in which to empty catheters and that there was poor attention to hand washing. Nosocomial transmission of infection is considered important in individuals with hospital-related UTIs, particularly those with urinary catheters (Gantz and Noskin, 1997).

Table 14.2: Characteristics of bacteria that cause catheter-associated urinary tract infections (UTIs)

Bacteria	Normal site	Biofilm formation	Pili	Gram stain	Survival in moist hospital environment	Associated with catheter blockage	Other comments
Escherichia coli	Intestinal tract	Yes	Yes	Negative			Produces toxins
Klebsiella oxytoca	External genital tract	Yes		Negative			Often found in patients who have been treated with antibiotics
Klebsiella pneumoniae	External genital tract	Yes		Negative antibiotics	Yes	No	treated with antibiotics
Proteus mirabilis	Distal urethra, intestinal tract	Yes	Yes	Negative		Yes	Urease producer, associated with alkaline urine, encrustation and stone formation
Pseudomonas aeruginosa	Intestinal tract, skin	Yes		Negative	Yes		Often associated with recurrent UTIs in hospital
Enterococcus faecalis	Intestinal tract			Negative			
Providencia stuartii	Intestinal tract	Yes		Negative	Yes	Yes	
Serratia marcescens	Intestinal tract			Negative	Yes		Often associated with recurrent UTIs in hospital
Diphtheroids	Skin	Yes		Positive			
Staphylococcus saprophyticus	Intestinal tract, skin			Positive			
Staphylococcus epidermidis	External genital tract, skin	Yes		Positive			
Streptococcus faecalis	Intestinal tract			Positive			

Characteristics described in the table are based on those stated in the identified sources; the gaps indicate where the information was not available. Source: Kunin (1989), Ramsay *et al* (1989), Shanson (1989), Murray *et al* (1990), Gould (1994), Ramirez De Arrellano *et al* (1994), Sleigh and Timbury (1994), Higgins (1995), Gantz and Noskin (1997), Morris *et al* (1997).

Complications of urinary tract infections

Catheter-associated UTIs are linked not only to morbidity but also mortality (Kunin *et al*, 1992). Occasionally, UTIs may reach the bloodstream causing septicaemia which is associated with a high rate of mortality (Wilson, 1997). Other complications of catheter-associated UTIs include pain and discomfort, leakage and bypassing of urine and blockage due to encrustation (Ramsay *et al*, 1989; Roe, 1993; Getliffe, 1996; Winson, 1997). It appears that *Proteus spp.* and other urease-producing micro-organisms play a key part in the formation of struvite by hydrolysing urea to ammonia (Kunin, 1989; Morris *et al*, 1997).

While some suggest that alkaline urine is associated with the formation of encrustations and subsequent blockage by precipitation of struvite crystals, others consider that the presence of pathogens which produce urease are not invariably associated with alkaline urine and precipitation of crystal (Hedelin *et al*, 1991). Encrustation appears to depend on individual factors including diet, urinary composition and catheter material (Burr and Nuseibeh, 1993; Roe, 1993; Winson, 1997). The formation of struvite bladder and kidney stones is linked to chronic infection (Griffith, 1978). Another complication of UTIs is the increased incidence of neoplastic changes in the bladder (Stickler and Zimakoff, 1994).

Implications for practice

Some characteristics of pathogenic bacteria associated with UTIs have been outlined. An important characteristic of certain bacteria is that they have the ability to form biofilms. Biofilms are implicated in encrustation, catheter blockage and urinary tract infections. The potential routes and sources of infection have also been described. A knowledge and understanding of the bacteriology discussed is necessary for informed nursing care and optimal catheter management. Key aspects of catheter management which minimise the incidence and complication of UTIs have been discussed elsewhere (Godfrey and Evans, 2000), but the principles of catheter care related to infection control are restated in *Table 14.3*.

Conclusion

A knowledge of the microbiology of catheter-associated UTIs should be the basis for determining the effective management of long-term indwelling urinary catheters. There is still a need to ensure that catheter care is based on evidence from clinical studies. The challenge is to minimise the incidence of catheter-associated UTIs and to limit the complications of such infections.

Table 14.3: Principles of catheter care to minimise incidence of urinary tract infections
Maintain a high fluid intake
Wash hands before and after emptying catheter bag
Use new gloves when emptying catheter bag
Empty catheter bag into a clean container
Wash perianal and meatal areas using soap and water
Change catheters according to manufacturer's recommendations
Change catheters proactively in individuals prone to catheter blockage
Maintain closed system and change bags at intervals of 5–7 days
Avoid using bladder washouts and instillations

Key points

❖ Urinary tract infection (UTI) associated with urinary catheterisation is the most common nosocomial infection.

❖ Many bacteria form a biofilm, a living layer of cells that stick to the surfaces of the catheter and catheter bag. Biofilms are associated with encrustation and catheter blockage.

❖ Complications of UTIs include pain and discomfort, leakage and bypassing of urine, blockage due to encrustation and, in some cases, raised mortality.

❖ A knowledge of microbiology provides a rationale for effective catheter care to minimise the incidence of catheter-associated UTIs.

References

Ayliffe G, Collins B, Taylor L (1991) *Hospital Acquired Infection: Principles and Prevention*. John Wright and Sons, London

Burr RG, Nuseibeh IM (1993) Blockage of indwelling urinary catheters: the roles of urinary composition, the catheter, medication and diet. *Paraplegia* 31: 234–41

Crow R, Chapman R, Roe B, Wilson J (1986) *A Study of Patients with an Indwelling Catheter and Related Nursing Practice*. Nursing Practice Research Unit, University of Surrey

Crumney V (1989) Ignorance can hurt. *Nurs Times* 85(21): 65–70

Gantz NM, Noskin GA (1997) Complicated UTI: targeting the pathogens. *Patient Care* 31(7): 212–6, 221–3

Getliffe K (1995) Long-term catheter use in the community. *Nurs Standard* 9(31): 25–7

Getliffe K (1996) Care of urinary catheters. *Nurs Standard* 11(11): 47–50

Getliffe K, Mulhall AB (1991) The encrustation of indwelling catheters. *Br J Urol* 67: 337–41

Godfrey H, Evans A (2000) Management of long-term urethral catheters: minimising complications. *Br J Nurs* 9(2): 74–81

Gould D (1994) Keeping on tract. *Nurs Times* 90(40): 58–63

Griffith DP (1978) Struvite stones. *Kidney Int* 13: 372–82

Hedelin H, Brah CG, Eckerdal G, Lincoln K (1991) Relationship between urease-producing, urinary pH and encrustation on indwelling urinary catheters. *Br J Urol* **67**: 527–31

Henry M (1992) Catheter confusion. *Nurs Times* **88**(42): 65–72

Higgins C (1995) Microbiological examination of urine in urinary tract infection. *Nurs Times* **91**(11): 33–5

Kennedy AP, Brocklehurst JC, Lye MDW (1983) Factors related to the problems of long-term catheterisation. *J Adv Nurs* **8**: 207–12

Khardori N, Yassien M (1995) Biofilms in device-related infections. *J Industrial Microbiol* **15**: 141–7

Kohler-Ockmore J, Feneley R (1996) Long-term catheterisation of the bladder: prevalence and morbidity. *Br J Urol* **77**: 347–51

Kunin CM (1989) Blockage of urinary catheters: role of micro-organisms and constituents of the urine on formation of encrustations. *J Clin Epidemiol* **42**(9): 835–42

Kunin CM, Douthitt S, Daning J, Anderson J, Moeschberger M (1992) The association between the use of urinary catheters and morbidity and mortality among elderly patients in nursing homes. *Am J Epidemiol* **135**: 291–301

Lowthian P (1998) The dangers of long-term catheter drainage. *Br J Nurs* **7**(7): 366–79

Morris NS, Stickler DJ, Winters C (1997) Which indwelling urethral catheters resist encrustation by *Proteus mirabilis* biofilms? *Br J Urol* **80**: 58–63

Mulhall AB, Chapman RG, Crow RA (1988a) The acquisition of bacteriuria. *Nurs Times* **84**(4): 61–2

Mulhall AB, Chapman RG, Crow RA (1988b) Bacteriuria during indwelling urethral catheterisation. *J Hosp Infection* **11**: 253–62

Mulhall AB (1991) Biofilms and urethral catheter infections. *Nurs Standard* **5**(18): 26–8

Murray PR, Drew WL, Kobayashi GS, Thompson JH (1990) *Medical Microbiology.* Wolfe Publishing, London

Parker LJ (1999) Urinary catheter management: minimising the risk of infection. *Br J Nurs* **8**(9): 563–74

Pinkerman ML (1994) Indwelling urinary catheters: reducing infection risks. *Nursing* **24**(9): 66, 68

Ramsay JWA, Garnham AJ, Mulhall AB, Crow RA, Bryan JM, Eardley I, Vale JA, Whitfield HN (1989) Biofilms, bacteria and bladder catheters: a clinical study. *Br J Urol* **64**: 395–98

Ramirez De Arrellano E, Pascual A, Martinez-Martinez L, Perea EJ (1994) Activity of eight antibacterial agents on *Staphylococcus epidermidis* attached to Teflon catheters. *J Med Microbiol* **40**: 43–7

Roe B (1993) Catheter-associated urinary tract infection: a review. *J Clin Nurs* **2**: 197–203

Shanson DC (1989) *Microbiology in Clinical Practice.* 2nd edn. Wright, London

Sleigh JD, Timbury MC (1994) *Notes on Medical Bacteriology.* 4th edn. Churchill Livingstone, Edinburgh

Smith H (1995) How bacteria cause disease. *Biol Sciences Rev* **7**(3): 2–6

Stickler D (1996) Bacterial biofilms and the encrustation of urethral catheters. *Biofouling* **9**(4): 293–305

Stickler D, Zimakoff J (1994) Complications of urinary tract infections associated with devices used for long- term bladder management. *J Hosp Infection* **20**: 177–94

Willis J (1995) Catheters urinary tract infections. *Nurs Times* **91**(35): 48–9

Wilson J (1997) Control and prevention of infection in catheter care. *Nurse Prescriber/Community Nurse* **3**(5): 39–40

Winn C (1996) Catheterisation: extending the scope of practice. *Nurs Standard* **10**(52): 49–54

Winson L (1997) Catheterisation: a need for improved patient management. *Br J Nurs* **6**(21): 1229–32

Woollons I (1996) Urinary catheters for long-term use. *Profess Nurse* **11**(12): 825–32

15

Urinary catheter management: minimising the risk of infection

Lynn J Parker

With catheterisation comes the risk of infection and therefore people should not be catheterised unless their clinical condition dictates that it is absolutely necessary. Nurses are responsible for both inserting catheters and the subsequent management of the catheterised patient. A high level of nursing knowledge and skill is required to achieve effective and safe management. This chapter continues the infection reviews the principles of catheter management with regard to controlling infection.

Catheterisation of patients both in hospital and the community is a common nursing procedure. An estimated 10–12% of patients in hospital (Crow *et al*, 1996) and 4% of community patients (Getliffe, 1990) have a urinary catheter *in situ* at any one time. At its most basic level a catheter is a hollow tube used to drain fluid from or put fluid into a body cavity. Urethral catheters are designed to be inserted into the bladder to assist in the drainage of urine, help with problems of incontinence, the instillation of treatments and for investigations (*Table 15.1*).

Table 15.1: Most common reasons for catheterisation	
Drainage of urine	Relief of acute or chronic urinary obstruction
	Emptying a hypotonic bladder
	Where sphincter dyssynergia prevents voiding
Incontinence	Last method of choice in the management of irreversible incontinence
Treatment	Pre- and post-surgical procedures
	Bladder irrigation, eg. by three-way drainage
	Cytotoxic therapy for papillary carcinoma
Investigations	To obtain uncontaminated specimens of urine
	To measure urinary output accurately, eg. in intensive care units
	To measure post-micturition urine volumes
	Urodynamic investigations
	X-ray investigations
Source: Pomfret (1996)	

The major problem associated with catheterisation is urinary tract infection (UTI). It has been found that hospital patients who are catheterised have significant levels of bladder bacteriuria within 72 hours (Crow *et al*, 1988) which are estimated to increase by 5–8% a day as long as the catheter remains *in situ* (Mulhall *et al*, 1988). The decision to catheterise, therefore, should only be taken after the implications and risks of the procedure have been carefully considered.

Complications may be reduced if the patient and his/her requirements are comprehensively assessed. Assessment should include the following information: the reason for catheterisation; the patient's medical and urological history; current health status; and any underlying conditions. This information ensures that the most suitable type of catheter is used and will give an indication of the type of complications to which the patient is vulnerable. Kohler-Ockmore (1993) described a programme of catheter management for people with long-term catheters; however, the principles can be applied to anyone who has to undergo this procedure.

Urinary tract infection

Emmerson *et al* (1996) found that 23.2% of hospital-acquired infections were in the urinary tract. In 1993, Falkiner listed the reasons as to why catheterised patients developed UTIs (*Table 15.2*).

In a non-catheterised patient the diagnosis of UTI is usually based on clinical symptoms which include frequency of micturition, pain on micturition (dysuria), fever and sometimes loin or suprapubic pain. These symptoms are the result of inflammation of the bladder or kidneys; in elderly people confusion can also be an indication of UTI. With regard to catheterisation, complications include significant bacteriuria, sepsis with significant patient mortality, urethral strictures, pressure necrosis, encrustation, block-

Table 15.2: Reasons why catheterised patients develop urinary tract infections
The catheter is a foreign body
It interferes with the normal process of urine excretion and the continual flushing effect
The catheterised bladder becomes a continuous culture apparatus with the reservoir of urine in the bladder (approximately 20ml is left, despite continuous draining) continually reinoculating the bladder with urethral and other organisms
Biofilms form on the surface of catheters that have been inserted for a period of time. These interfere with effective antibiotic therapy or antiseptic washouts
Source: Falkiner (1993)

age, bypassing and spasm (Stickler and Zimakoff, 1994).

The nurse should observe the urine when emptying the catheter drainage bag for amount and colour: cloudy urine and a distinct fishy smell are indications of UTI. Urine itself is a sterile fluid and the laboratory may confirm diagnosis by the isolation of 10^5 organisms/ml from a specimen of urine. White blood cells in the urine provide evidence of the inflammatory process, which may be caused by infection. Bacteriuria occurs when bacteria colonise the urinary tract without invading the tissues and is normally associated with catheterisation; colonisation frequently disappears after the catheter is removed.

Stickler and Zimakoff (1994), in a 12-month study of device-related UTIs, found that in comparison with non-catheterised patients, patients with long-term indwelling catheters in nursing homes were three times more likely to receive antibiotics, three times more likely to be hospitalised and three times more likely to be dead at the end of the year.

Choice of catheter materials

Today, many types of catheters are available. Evidence exists that as far back as the third century BC rigid metal tubes, either straight or curved, with a hole at the tip, were used as catheters (Bloom *et al*, 1994). However, these types of tubes caused trauma to the patient. By the end of the nineteenth century, following the vulcanisation of rubber in 1844 (Marino *et al*, 1993), durable and flexible catheters were widely used. During the 1900s, new plastic materials became available: silicone, Teflon coatings and polyvinylchloride (PVC). However, latex catheters remain the popular choice of the day for short-term use (Woodward, 1997).

Catheters are described as short-term when they are changed between 14 and 28 days, and long-term if they remain in place for up to 12 weeks. The proposed length of use should guide the nurse in his/her choice of catheter. General recommendations are that uncoated latex catheters should be avoided but that Teflon-coated latex catheters are acceptable for the short-term. Silicone, silicone elastomer-coated latex and hydrogel-coated latex are acceptable for longer-term use (Sutton, 1992). Latex catheters have been associated with a variety of infection complications (Cox *et al*, 1989), encrustation (Cox *et al* 1987; Getliffe and Mulhall, 1991) and cytotoxicity (Ruutu *et al*, 1985).

All catheters currently have to pass safety standards devised by the British Standard Committee (British Standard Institute 1695, 1990a,b). In the UK, these relate to cytotoxicity tests for medical rubber and plastics and are concerned with catheters' base format and coated format where applicable.

Finally, it is worth considering the catheters which the ward stocks, as this will guide the choice of catheter, and how catheters are stored. For example, an audit looking at ward stock levels found that 65.7% of wards possessed stock that was more than five years old and that damage to the catheter packaging, and potential damage due to direct heat or sunlight, was recorded in several areas (Mulhall and Lee, 1990). The easiest way to store catheters is in the manufacturers' boxes, which should be clearly labelled and kept away from direct heat or sunlight. Local policies should be drawn up by expert personnel to guide staff in relation to the selection, ordering and stock control of catheters.

Types of catheterisation

The two methods of urethral catheterisation are intermittent or indwelling.

Intermittent catheterisation

Intermittent catheterisation involves periodically inserting a single channel catheter into the bladder. This is usually for the relief of urinary retention but it may also be used to give medication intravesically (Pomfret, 1996). Patients are usually taught to do this procedure themselves using a clean as opposed to an aseptic technique. However, many patients who would benefit from using this technique are not given the opportunity to do so because healthcare professionals lack knowledge in this area (Haynes, 1994).

Indwelling catheters

Indwelling catheters are held in position by an inflated balloon (Winson, 1997) (*Figure 15.1*). They were developed in the 1930s by Dr Frederic B Foley and are therefore known as Foley catheters. They can be inserted into the bladder by the natural channel of the urethra or through a suprapubic incision.

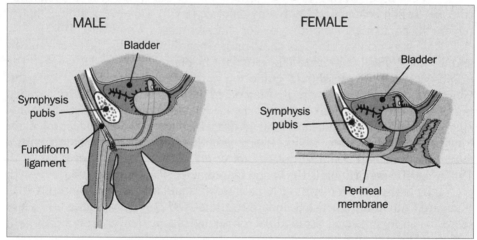

Figure 15.1: Diagrams showing male and female catheters in position in the bladder

The suprapubic route (*Figure 15.2*) is increasing in use because of its perceived advantages: ease of re-catheterisation; no trauma to the urethra; less obstruction for sexual activity; and greater patient comfort (Iacovou, 1994). There is a lower density of bacteria on the abdominal skin and therefore it is thought that this results in a lower incidence of bacteriuria than that associated with urethral catheters. However, evidence suggests that while the onset of infection may be delayed, prolonged drainage via a suprapubic catheter inevitably results

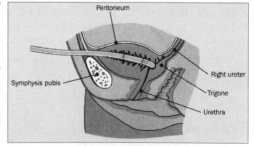

Figure 15.2: Diagram showing a catheter inserted by the suprapubic route

in bacteriuria. Other problems include blockage of the catheter and formation of bladder calculi (Stickler and Zimakoff, 1994).

Unlike intermittent catheterisation, which is a clean technique, the insertion of indwelling catheters, either by the urethral or suprapubic route, requires an aseptic technique if performed by the nurse.

Aspects of care

Choosing a system

Until recently little choice was available to nurses in relation to the the type of indwelling or intermittent catheter they could use. Although the choice is wider today, a study in 1982 showed that nurses lacked knowledge in relation to what catheters were available and when they could be most appropriately used (Kennedy and Brocklehurst, 1982). Catheterisation is an embarrassing and sometimes a traumatic experience and therefore patients rely on nurses for support and advice.

The first question to ask is whether the catheter needs to be of the indwelling variety. Some patients may be suitable candidates for intermittent self-catheterisation; this will depend on their level of dexterity and determination to manage this area of care. Consideration should be given to the length of time that the catheter will remain *in situ* and whether the suprapubic or urethral route is the best option.

Catheter size is measured in Charrière (Ch) (internal diameter measurements) or French gauge (Fg) units (outer circumference). A 12Ch catheter easily allows drainage of normal volumes of urine. Most catheters have a 10ml balloon capacity. Large balloons were originally designed to reduce postoperative haemorrhage; 30ml balloons still exist but they are not recommended for general use as they tend to sit higher in the bladder allowing residual urine to collect under the balloon (Winson, 1997), which then becomes a reservoir for infection (*Figure 15.3*).

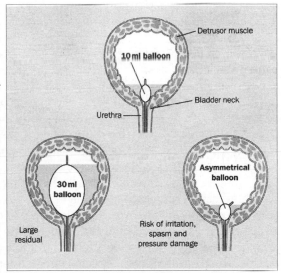

Figure 15.3: Positions of balloons in the bladder

Large catheters and balloons are associated with increased bladder irritability which causes painful spasms and leakage (Kennedy *et al*, 1983). They also block the urethral glands and because of pressure cause ulceration of the bladder neck. The recommended size is 12–16Ch for women and 14–16Ch for men, with a 10ml balloon. These sizes are sufficient to allow adequate drainage of urine from the average person in a 24-hour period; smaller sizes are available for children (*Table 15.3*).

Table 15.3: Choosing a system	
Duration	Short-term (1–28 days): latex, PVC, Teflon-coated. Long-term (>12 weeks): silicone, silicone-elastomer coated latex, hydrogel-coated latex.
Size	Male 14–46 Ch; length 41cm (average) Female 12–14 Ch; length 23cm (average)
Balloon size	5–10ml routine 30ml (surgery only)
Adapted from: Winson (1997); PVC=polyvinylchloride	

For female catheterisation specific female catheters exist that have a shorter shaft length of 23cm as opposed to male catheters which are 41cm in length. These shorter catheters, although not suitable for all women, allow more efficient drainage by reducing the risk of looping and kinking; they also reduce the risk of upward gradient drainage of the tube (Wright, 1991). They can also be discreetly concealed, if used in conjunction with a leg bag, on the mid-thigh below the skirt hemline. Problems of traction and pulling upon the bladder neck occur if the leg drainage bag is not adequately secured. Also, some obese women complain that the balloon inflation valve is uncomfortable and rubs between their thighs (Wright, 1991).

The choice of drainage system is also important. This is dictated by the patient and the reason for the catheterisation. It has long been recognised that using a closed-drainage system can dramatically reduce the incidence of catheter-acquired UTI (Kunin, 1980). The importance of a closed-drainage system was demonstrated in a study by Garibaldi *et al* (1974) which demonstrated that bacteriuria increased when the catheter tubing junction was open, the drainage bag was improperly positioned, or the drainage spigot was unclamped. This latter fact resulted in the drainage bag spigot being replaced by the outlet tap.

Another study showed that disconnecting the catheter from the drainage bag significantly increased infection rates (Platt *et al*, 1982). The drainage bag is considered to be a 'reservoir of potential pathogens' (Maizels and Schaeffer, 1980). Bacteria migrate along the lumen of the catheter from a contaminated drainage system; adding a disinfectant to the bag does not significantly reduce the incidence of infection in catheterised patients (Crow *et al*, 1988).

For short-term use and non-ambulatory patients, a single 1–2 litre drainage bag, with or without an outlet tap, supported on a stand on the floor or by a hanger on the bed frame, is recommended (Brown, 1992). For long-term use the emphasis should be on the patient's needs. The drainage bag can be supported by a holster suspended from a belt around the waist; alternatively, a smaller leg bag strapped to the thigh or calf during the day can be used. Some bags have a cloth backing for greater comfort when coming into contact with the skin. At night a bag with a larger volume can replace or be linked to the leg bag via the outlet tap.

Whether or not the catheter should be fixed to the leg continues to be a source of controversy as there is a lack of evidence on this point (Pomfret, 1991). The advice given is that the nurse should assess whether there is a risk of traction to the catheter and, if so, is the best suspension method being used, eg. holster or catheter strap. Adhesive materials should be avoided and care should be taken not to occlude the lumen or cause constriction to the limb (Pomfret, 1996).

An alternative to the leg bag is the catheter valve. This is attached to an indwelling catheter and enables the user to stop the flow of urine for periods of time (Doherty, 1999). Assessment is necessary to ensure that patients have enough dexterity to use the valve appropriately and bladder function also needs to be assessed. At present no research exists in relation to catheter valves and the risk of infection.

Nurses need to be aware of the key role they play in the management of maintaining a closed-drainage system and ensuring that breaks to the system are kept to an absolute minimum and are tailored to the patient's needs.

Catheter insertion

Attitudes towards male catheterisation have varied over the years. Historically, only doctors and male nurses catheterised men because it was felt that female nurses lacked knowledge of male anatomy; the aim was also to preserve male modesty and prevent embarrassment of female nurses when in close proximity to male genitalia (Courcy-Ireland, 1993). However, an increasing number of female nurses are now undertaking male catheterisation.

Unskilled practitioners can easily and unknowingly cause considerable pain and trauma, not only to the urethra but also to the bladder neck, if they are not fully aware of the risks involved in catheterisation.

Before inserting a catheter, the genitalia should be cleaned aseptically as they are normally colonised by skin and faecal organisms (Brown, 1992). Once the catheter has been selected it should be attached to an appropriate drainage bag to provide a closed system and inserted using an aseptic technique. Tissue damage can be minimised by careful insertion techniques and the use of an anaesthetic gel before catheterisation (Brown, 1992); this applies to women as well as men. Adequate lighting is also a necessity, especially when catheterising women; poor lighting can result in contamination as the catheter may inadvertently touch the surrounding area or it may be inserted into the vagina. If the latter occurs the catheter must be discarded as it is no longer sterile and the nurse must replace his/her gloves before inserting a new catheter (Horton and Parker, 1997). It is important that nurses wash their hands both before and after the procedure.

Meatal and perineal hygiene

Debate continues with regard to the value of undertaking meatal toilet. Common practice is that meatal toilet using an antiseptic lotion should be carried out every six hours. However, the research is inconclusive and does not support this practice as a means of preventing UTIs.

Washing with soap and water once daily, as part of the patient's daily hygiene for the genital area or as required on an individual patient care basis, and drying thoroughly is as effective as carrying out regular meatal toilet (Horton and Parker, 1997). If the catheter becomes encrusted around the urethra after daily bathing, then washing the area with soap and water as necessary is sufficient (Burke *et al*, 1981, 1983). While cleaning the catheter should not be pulled outwards as this can traumatise the urethra. Nurses must wash their hands before and after any catheter-related procedure.

Patients with catheters can bathe on a daily basis as studies have shown that water does not enter the bladder of patients with catheters during bathing (De Groot, 1979). For the patient's comfort it is recommended that the drainage bag is emptied before bathing.

Emptying the drainage bag

The emptying of patients' urinary drainage bags must not be part of a general round where nurses go from one catheterised patient to another emptying the bags, as this increases the risk of cross-infection (Glenister, 1987). Hands should be washed before and after handling the drainage bag and gloves should be worn to prevent contamination from body fluids. Patients should have their own containers; these can be either a single-use container, eg. a disposable urinal, or a jug that can be heat-disinfected. Brown (1992) states that the catheter tap should be cleaned with 70% alcohol before and after use; however, there is lack of evidence that cleaning the tap is effective in reducing the risk of infection. The nurse must ensure that the tap does not touch the sides of the container when the bag is being emptied. It is also suggested that the drainage bag is changed at the same time as the catheter is changed, or if it leaks or becomes contaminated (Brown, 1992).

Bladder washouts

Up to 50% of long-term catheterised patients suffer recurrent catheter blockage (Getliffe, 1994). This can be the result of bladder spasm, twisted tubing or constipation. However, the most common cause is the encrustation of the surface of the catheter with deposits of mineral salts from urine (Getliffe, 1996). The value of antiseptic bladder washouts for patients with long-term catheters is questionable as they can increase the risk of infection by breaking the closed system (Crow *et al*, 1988). However, bladder washouts containing Suby G or mandelic acid do dissolve encrustations. Not more than 50ml of solution should be retained for 15 minutes with at least 48 hours interval between washouts (Getliffe, 1996).

Reducing the alkalinity of the urine by taking oral agents such as cranberry juice requires further research. It is thought that cranberry juice has the ability to

acidify the urine to a level of pH5.5, so achieving and su
which helps in clearing UTIs (Leaver, 1996). However, larg
(1500–4000ml daily) or juice with a high concentration of cra
in order to achieve this outcome.

Fluid intake

Once a catheter has been inserted it is important that the patient mainta s an
adequate fluid intake. This helps in reducing the risk of constipation or the
irritant effect of concentrated urine on the bladder. An intake of between two and
three litres per day is advised as this will result in a dilute urine output and will
enable the use of smaller gauge catheters (Brown, 1992; Pomfret, 1996).

Clamping of catheters

Historically, catheters have always been clamped before their removal to assess
bladder tone (Pomfret, 1996); however, there is no evidence to support this
action. In practice the clamps are often forgotten and left on the catheter leaving
the bladder to fill with urine, so increasing the risk of infection.

Taking specimens

Urine specimens must never be taken from the drainage bag. They must always
be taken from the sample port as described in local policies. Also, the catheter
must not be disconnected from the drainage bag to obtain specimens.

Removing the catheter

The longer a catheter remains *in situ* the higher the risk of the patient acquiring a
UTI; consequently, catheters should be removed at the earliest opportunity. The
risk of infection in suprapubic and intermittent urethral catheters is lower than in
urethral catheters (Warren, 1991) (see also 'indwelling catheters' section). The
perineal area is heavily contaminated with micro-organisms, especially faecal
organisms such as *Escherichia coli* which are associated with UTIs. While
intermittent catheters may introduce a number of micro-organisms on insertion,
the patient's immune system should be able to counteract these as they are few in
number and the catheter does not remain permanently in the bladder.

Patient information

Education about catheters has been shown to have a significant effect on
patients' acceptance of their catheter. Information leaflets are freely available
from manufacturers. Nurses need to be sensitive when helping people establish
good patterns for managing their catheters. Roe (1991) showed that patients and
carers need to be encouraged to maintain high standards of hygiene.

Roe and Brocklehurst (1987) showed that professionals did not discuss sex with patients who had been catheterised. There are no links between sexual activity, catheters and infection. The emphasis should be on personal hygiene and patient education. *Table 15.4* lists the points that catheterised patients need to consider in relation to sexual activity. Patients must be encouraged to participate actively with regard to the options that are available to them.

Table 15.4: Advice regarding sexual activity and catheters
Catheters do not have to be removed before making love
In men, once an erection is achieved the catheter can be taped back or a condom used as this should not cause irritation to the partner. However, it may be more traumatic to the urethra and therefore suprapubic catheters may be more appropriate for sexually active people
Women should be told where their catheter is inerted so that they know it is not in the vagina; the catheter can be strapped onto the abdomen
The 'missionary' position can cause tension on catheters so trial and error is needed in relation to positioning
KY Jelly can be used to increase lubrication
Catheterised patients can be shown how to remove and reinsert their catheter before and after intercourse
Patients should be told what counselling is available to them
Source: Britton and Wright (1990); Atkinson (1997)

Conclusion

Nurses have a central role in the care of patients with a urinary drainage system. Studies suggest that there is a lack of knowledge in selecting equipment and attention needs to be directed at nursing procedures. It is important that all aspects of care relating to catheterisation have a scientific basis and that this is reflected in the education and training of nurses.

Key points

❖ Catheterisation is a common procedure for 10–12% of hospital patients and 4% of community patients.

❖ A major risk of catheterisation is the development of urinary tract infection.

❖ Criteria should exist for choosing the appropriate catheter and drainage system to meet the needs of individual patients.

❖ Patients should be involved in all aspects of catheter care.

❖ Use of analgesic gel, for women as well as men, before catheter insertion, reduces pain, facilitates ease of access to the urethra and can reduce infection rates.

❖ There is a lack of knowledge among healthcare professionals in the selection and management of urinary drainage systems.

References

Atkinson K (1997) Incorporating sexual health into catheter care. *Prof Nurse* **13**(3): 146–8

Bloom DA, McGuire EJ, Lapides J (1994) A brief history of urethral catheterisation. *J Urol* **151**: 317–25

British Standard Institute 1695 (1990a) *Urological Catheters: Part 1. Specification for Sterile, Single-use Urethral Catheters of the Nelaton and Foley Types.* The Stationery Office, London

British Standard Institute 1695 (1990b) *Urological Catheters: Part 2. Specification for Sterile, Single-use Urethral Catheters of the Tiemann, Whistle Tip, 3-way and Haematuria Types.* The Stationery Office, London

Britton PM, Wright E (1990) Nursing care of catheterised patients. *Prof Nurse* **5**(6): 231–4

Brown M (1992) Urinary catheters: patient management. *Nurs Standard* **6**(19): 29–31

Burke JP, Garibaldi RA, Britt MR, Jacobson JA, Conti M, Alling DW (1981) Prevention of catheter-associated urinary tract infections. Efficacy of daily meatal care regimens. *Am J Med* **70**: 655–8

Burke JP, Jacobson JA, Garibaldi RA, Conti M, Alling DW (1983) Evaluation of daily meatal care with poly-antibiotic ointment in the prevention of urinary catheter associated bacteriuria. *J Urol* **129**: 331–4

Courcy-Ireland K (1993) An issue of sensitivity: use of analgesic gel in catheterising women. *Prof Nurse* **8**(11): 738–42

Cox AJ, Harries JE, Hukins DWL *et al* (1987) Calcium phosphate in catheter encrustation. *Br J Urol* **59**(2): 159–63

Cox AJ, Hukins DWL, Sutton TM (1989) Infection of catheterised patients: bacterial colonization of encrusted Foley catheters shown by scanning electron microscopy. *Urol Res* **17**(6): 349–52

Crow RA, Chapman RG, Roe B, Wilson J (1996) *A Study of Patients with an Indwelling Catheter and Related Nursing Practice.* Nursing Practice Research Unit, University of Surrey

Crow RA, Mulhall A, Chapman R (1988) Indwelling catheterisation and related nursing practice. *J Adv Nurs* **13**: 489–95

De Groot JE (1979) Entrance of H_2O into the bladder during bathing in elderly catheterised and non-catheterised females. *Investigative Urol* **17**(3): 207–9

Doherty W (1999) The Sims Portex Catheter Valve: an alternative to the leg bag. *Br J Nurs* **8**(7): 459–62

Emmerson AM, Enstone JE, Griffin M, Kelsey MC, Smyth ETM (1996) The second prevalence survey of infection in hospitals — overview of the results. *J Hosp Infection* **32**: 175–90

Falkiner FR (1993) The insertion and management of indwelling urethral catheters — minimising the risk of infection. *J Hosp Infection* **25**: 79–90

Garibaldi RA, Burke JP, Dickman ML, Smith CB (1974) Factors predisposing to bacteriuria during indwelling urethral catheterisation. *N Engl J Med* **291**(5): 215–19

Getliffe K (1990) Catheter blockage in community patients. *Nurs Standard* **5**(9): 33–6

Getliffe KA, Mulhall AB (1991) The encrustation of indwelling catheters. *Br J Urol* **67**(4): 337–41

Getliffe KA (1994) The use of bladder washouts to reduce urinary catheter encrustation. *J Urol* **73**: 696–700

Getliffe KA (1996) Bladder instillations and washouts in the management of catheter patients. *J Adv Nurs* **23**: 548–54

Glenister H (1987) The passage of infection. *Nurs Times* **83**(22): 68–73

Haynes A (1994) Intermittent self-catheterisation — the key facts. *Prof Nurse* **10**(2): 100–4

Horton R, Parker LJ (1997) *Informed Infection Control Practice.* Churchill Livingstone, New York

Iacovou JW (1994) Suprapubic catheterisation of the urinary bladder. *Hospital Update* **20**(3): 159–62

Kennedy AP, Brocklehurst JC (1982) The nursing management of patients with long-term indwelling catheters. *J Adv Nurs* **7**: 411

Kennedy AP, Brocklehurst JC, Lye MDW (1983) Factors related to the problems of long-term catheterisation. *J Adv Nurs* **8**: 207–12

Kohler-Ockmore J (1993) Catheter concerns. *Nurs Times* **89**(2): 34–6

Kunin CM (1980) Urinary tract infections. In symposium on surgical infection. *Surg Clin Am* **60**: 223–31

Leaver RB (1996) Cranberry juice. *Prof Nurse* **11**(8): 525–6

Marino RA, Mooppan UMM, Kim H (1993) History of urethral catheters and their balloons: drainage, anchorage, dilation and haemostasis. *J Endourology* **7**(2): 89–92

Maizels M, Schaeffer AJ (1980) Decreased incidence of bacteriuria associated with periodic instillations of hydrogen peroxide into the urethral catheter drainage bag. *J Urol* **123**: 841–5

Mulhall AB, Lee K (1990) The provision of urethral catheters: an equipment audit. *Quality Assurance in Health Care* **2**(2): 145–8

Mulhall AB, Chapman RG, Crow RA (1988) Bacteriuria during indwelling urethral catheterisation. *J Hosp Infection* **11**: 253–62

Platt R, Polk BF, Murdock B, Rosner B (1982) Mortality associated with nosocomial urinary tract infection. *N Engl J Med* **307**(11): 637–41

Pomfret I (1991) The catheter debate. *Nurs Times* **87**(37): 67–8

Pomfret I (1996) Catheters: design, selection and management. *Br J Nurs* **5**(4): 245–51

Roe BH (1991) Study of the effects of education on the management of urine drainage systems by patients and carers. *J Adv Nurs* **15**: 223–31

Roe BH, Brocklehurst JC (1987) Study of patients with indwelling catheters. *J Adv Nurs* **12**: 713–19

Ruutu M, Alfthan O, Talja M, Anderson LC (1985) Cytotoxicity of latex urinary catheters. *Br J Urol* **57**(1): 82–7

Stickler DJ, Zimakoff J (1994) Complications of urinary tract infections associated with devices used for long-term bladder management. *J Hospital Infection* **28**: 177–94

Sutton T (1992) Material benefits. *Nurs Times* **88**(31): 62

Warren JW (1991) The catheter and urinary tract infection. *Med Clin North Am* **75**(2): 481–93

Winson L (1997) Catheterisation: a need for improved patient management. *Br J Nurs* **6**(21): 1229–52

Woodward S (1997) Complications of allergies to latex catheters. *Br J Nurs* **6**(14): 786–93

Wright ES (1991) A choice to help meet women's needs: developments in female urethral catheters. *Prof Nurse* **6**(4): 226–8

Section four
Perspectives of education, research and audit

16

Educational preparation: specialist practice in continence care

KS Williams, RP Assassa, NKG Smith, C Shaw and E Carter

Contributing factors to effective continence service provision include funding, organisation and expert knowledge among the individuals providing care. Expert knowledge can be gained through clinical experience and appropriate ongoing education. It has been widely reported that undergraduate education in this area for nurses, doctors and physiotherapists is limited (Brocklehurst, 1990; Swaffield, 1994; Laycock, 1995). Many nurses providing continence care have accumulated knowledge through experience and trial and error. Little is known about the effectiveness of advanced postgraduate education of 'experts' in continence care. This chapter outlines a continence education module developed to prepare a specialist group of nurses to provide a high standard of continence care that is both safe and effective in a clinical environment. This module was designed and evaluated specifically as part of the Leicestershire Medical Research Council (MRC) Incontinence Study. Changes in continence knowledge, attitudes to research, and acceptability of the module have been explored. When setting up a new nurse-led continence service, it is of great importance to systematically detail the components of the educational preparation of the nurses providing the service. Open discussion of any problems in the design and implementation of this module may inform future modules in this and other areas.

Incontinence is a major problem with an estimated 2% of the UK population needing services (Perry *et al*, 1999). Services can be provided in a number of ways, but almost always include a designated nursing input. It is well documented that UK continence services have developed in a largely ad hoc manner (Royal College of Physicians, 1995; Roe *et al*, 1996). Similarly, educational preparation of continence nurses has been provided, with the English National Board (ENB) 978 course usually being the only required education for nurses specialising in continence provision.

The ENB course is a well established short course delivered at local level, but it is based on a centrally (ENB) generated outline curriculum. Although the course is validated by the Board, it is open to criticism due to inconsistencies in delivery pattern, variation in its interpretation, and its basic level of instruction.

Such courses are difficult to standardise. Rhodes and Parker (1993) reported that continence advisers recognised the need for an advanced course as a means of strengthening their role, and enhancing their professional credibility, in addition to providing them with the necessary skills to fulfil their role.

In more recent years, with the move towards nursing preparation in higher education, some universities have developed undergraduate continence modules. The ENB A57 course offers one model of how such education programmes can be delivered; it uses a modular approach and includes four separate modules covering clinical practice, health promotion and bowel dysfunction as well as an introductory module. However, its availability is extremely limited (ENB course A57, basic course outline).

The purpose of this chapter is to describe an education module designed to prepare nurses to work as continence nurse practitioners (CNPs) in a service developed as part of a research study. This model of education provision has been fully evaluated and while not exhaustive in its coverage may go some way to providing a core module for future continence programmes.

As part of a study, funded by the Medical Research Council (MRC), which is currently being carried out, entitled 'Incontinence — a population laboratory approach to the epidemiology and evaluation of care', a randomised controlled trial of two types of service provision for the management of urinary and faecal incontinence is being undertaken. Comparison is being made between existing services in Leicestershire, which centre on the primary healthcare team, and the new study service which centres on CNPs working in the community with support from both GPs and a hospital medical team.

The CNP service consists of assessment, investigation and diagnosis of people with urinary symptoms. On the basis of the assessment, CNPs implement primary interventions which include:

- bladder re-education
- pelvic floor awareness
- bulbar massage for post-micturition dribble
- treatment of candidiasis, atrophic vaginitis, and urinary tract infection.

CNPs also offer advice on diet, fluid intake, and incomplete bladder emptying. Patients who fail to respond to these primary interventions are offered secondary interventions by the CNP for the treatment of genuine stress incontinence and detrusor instability (*Table 16.1*).

Table 16.1: Expertise offered by the continence nurse practitioner service
Nursing assessment
Institution of information and appropriate investigations
Symptomatic diagnosis
Comprehensive treatment and follow-up
Continuation of patient care across primary and secondary care boundaries
Performance and interpretation of the advanced diagnostic technique of urodynamics

The CNP is the essential component of the new service and as such his/her preparation for the role is crucial. This chapter documents the educational preparation of CNPs, in both theory and practice, and evaluates the education programme in terms of continence knowledge, and attitudes to research, as well as expectations of and satisfaction with the module.

The continence module

The aim was to provide a specialised, professionally relevant programme of academic study building on nurses' existing experience, skills and knowledge. A three-month module was developed to provide a thorough grounding in the theory and practice of care and treatment of adults with incontinence. The objectives of the module are detailed in *Table 16.2.*

Table 16.2: Module objectives	
Integrate theoretical and clinical skills to:	Independently assess individuals with UD
	Independently diagnose individuals with UD
Demonstrate discrimination and analytical skills in problem solving when:	Investigating individuals with UD
	Treating individuals with UD
	Monitoring individuals with UD
Incorporate theoretical/practical knowledge to:	Effectively carry out urodynamic investigation
	Interpret urodynamic findings
Demonstrate a high standard of client/carer interaction rooted in knowledge of the psychosocial needs of clients	
Advance nursing practice through the application of specialist skills related to UD	
Critically evaluate the contribution of research to clinical practice and demonstrate a sound knowledge of the research questions being asked within the study	
UD=urinary dysfunction	

The module was accredited at level three by De Montfort University, Leicester, within an undergraduate programme of study. The three-month programme consisted of 120 sessions of three hours duration, 50% of which comprised theoretical teaching and 50% practical teaching. The programme of study ran full-time. The structure of the module was designed to enable students to practise safely, using knowledge based on current research evidence.

A number of teaching methods were used, including a total of 30 class contact sessions, six tutorials, 30 practical sessions, and 14 self-directed-learning sessions. The module was run from a classroom on a general hospital site with access to clinical and teaching equipment. The students had easy access to university and hospital library facilities. A module management team was responsible for the efficient and effective operation of the programme. The programme was taught by a multidisciplinary team comprising nurses, physiotherapists, gynaecologists, urologists, health psychologists, epidemiologists, statisticians, and gerontologists.

Five key areas were covered within the module relating to theory and practice:

1. Formulating a diagnosis through accurate assessment.
2. Provision of appropriate treatment.
3. Technical skills.
4. Research skills.
5. Teamwork and interpersonal skills.

Within each of these broad key areas, a number of subjects were covered (*Table 16.3*).

Table 16.3: Module content	
Formulating a diagnosis through accurate assessment	Anatomy and physiology: normal micturition Aetiology: factors which cause or worsen incontinence Clinical skills: medical assessment, clinical history, nursing assessment, history taking, diary keeping, pad tests Examination skills: physical examination
Provision of appropriate treatment	Nursing treatment of incontinence, eg. bladder re-education, fluid and diet advice Physiotherapy: principles, limitations and practical application of pelvic floor therapies Urology: indications for conservative and surgical interventions Surgery: benefits, limitations and complications of surgery Drug therapy: indications, benefits and limitations of antibiotics, oestrogen therapy, anticholinergics and iatrogenic causes of incontinence Service provision: need for continence services
Technical skills	Urodynamics: theory and practical application Interpretation of urodynamic investigation Phlebotomy
Research skills	Principles of research and critical appraisal skills Application of research to clinical practice
Teamwork, interpersonal skills, professional issues	Time management: prioritisation of tasks Patient/carer education, eg. identification of patient/carer educational needs Legal/ethical implications, eg. medico-legal issues associated with the continence nurse practitioner role

Information relating to each of the subjects covered was detailed in a curriculum document indicating rationale, aim, learning objectives, teaching and learning strategies, proposed delivery pattern (theory and practice), and assessment. In addition, a student handbook was provided detailing relevant information taken from the curriculum document.

Two 3000-word essays were required from students for assessment purposes. Keeping a reflective journal was encouraged throughout the module (UKCC, 1996). This module formed part of an ongoing programme of continuing education which has, to date, covered urodynamics theory, practice and inter-pretation, and the practical and theoretical teaching of pelvic floor therapies and their assessment.

Evaluation of the module

Having described the education module this chapter will assess its effectiveness in terms of improving nurses' knowledge.

The aims of the evaluation were as follows:

- to measure the change in nurses' knowledge of incontinence pre- and post-module
- to measure the change in nurses' attitudes towards research pre- and post-module
- to explore to what extent nurses' expectations of the module were achieved.

Methods

The study adopted a simple pre- and post-test approach. A questionnaire using both open-ended questions and fixed responses was adopted and administered at the commencement of the module and three months later at its completion. In addition, semi-structured interviews were tape-recorded after completion of the programme.

Six nurses, each having a minimum of three years postregistration experience, undertook the programme. Two comparison groups (historical controls) were used to examine the representativeness of the newly recruited CNPs. These were drawn from nurses involved in a previous study examining knowledge and attitudes towards incontinence. Control group 1 comprised 23 nurses and was used to compare pre-module knowledge scores. Control group 2 comprised nine nurses and was used to compare research attitude scores. The control groups and CNPs (ie. the experimental group) were comparable in terms of grade, qualifications and nursing experience.

A semi-structured questionnaire was used and included questions relating to definitions of incontinence and its epidemiology, the main types of incontinence, methods of assessing patients with incontinence, and strategies for the promotion of continence. The 'attitudes to research scale' was adapted from a previously derived scale. A qualitative methodology was also employed to explore expectations of and satisfaction with the module. Semi-structured tape-recorded interviews were carried out by an independent trained interviewer with the nurses' consent. Data were collected in the first week of the education programme and three weeks after its completion.

A total knowledge score of 47 could be achieved and a total research attitude score of 35 could be obtained from questions relating to attitudes towards research; a high score indicated a positive attitude towards research. The taped interviews were transcribed and the text for each interview labelled sequentially and numbered to identify sentences belonging to the subjects or the interviewer. Themes that arose in two or more of the interviews were identified and placed on a grid for ease of reference. The following areas were explored within the interviews:

- expectations of the module
- most important aspect of the module
- limitations of the education module.

Results

Knowledge of incontinence

The mean pre-module knowledge score for the CNP group was 18 (38%). This compared with a score of 11 (23%) in control group 1 out of a possible maximum score of 47 (*Figure 16.1*). All of the CNPs improved their knowledge scores (*Figure 16.2*). There was an overall improvement in knowledge score after undertaking the module from a mean of 18 (38%) to 25 (53%) (*t*-test, *P*=0.001) (*Figure 16.2*).

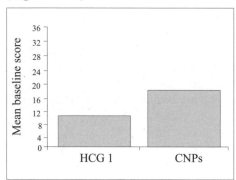

Figure 16.1: Mean baseline knowledge score. HCG=historical control group; CNP=continence nurse practitioner

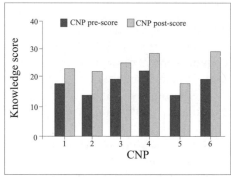

Figure 16.2: CNPs' incontinence knowledge pre- and post-module. CNP=continence nurse practitioner

Attitudes to research

The mean research attitude score for the CNP group pre-module was 28 (80%), which compared with 22 (63%) in control group 2 out of a possible score of 35 (*Figure 16.3*).

There was an overall improvement in research attitude scores after the module from a mean 28 (80%) to 30 (86%) (*Figure 16.4*).

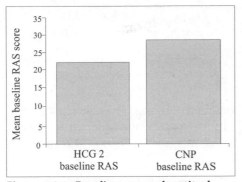

Figure 16.3: Baseline research attitude score (RAS). HCG=historical control group; CNP=continence nurse practitioner

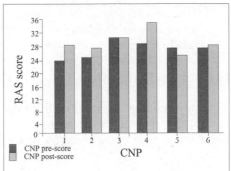

Figure 16.4: CNP research attitude score pre- and post-module. CNP=continence nurse practitioner; RAS=research attitude score

Taped interviews

Expectations of the module

Three of the nurses commented that the education programme was much as they had expected and two referred to the student handbook which had set out the content of the education programme and gave some idea of what to expect. One nurse stated that the education programme covered more than expected:

I think we did more than I expected us to do, a lot more, more at a higher level as well.

Two of the nurses did not have any expectations of the programme:

To be honest I didn't know what to expect!

Having established what expectations the CNP group had at the outset of the programme, this area was further explored by asking if their expectations had been met. Overall, the CNPs felt that their objectives had been met:

Well, educationally it did meet my objectives.

It covered pretty much everything and more.

However, there were some expectations reported which referred to the limits of the practical sessions which were available for the gaining of practical skills:

I expected more practical experience.

Most important part of the programme

When asked what was the most important aspect of the programme, the majority felt it was having obtained sufficient knowledge to undertake their role:

Coming out with the knowledge that I need to do the job, I think that's the most important one.

I think to me it was all important, because I knew that you had to take it all in to be able to ultimately go out there and just practise independently, so no there wasn't any one thing.

Limitations of the module

The limitations of the module from the perspective of the CNPs were explored. Again, the issue of insufficient practical clinical experience came up for two of the nurses. One nurse referred to the actual mix of the theory and practical sessions.

I think you need to mix practice and theory, but we found it just wasn't mixed evenly — one would go to a certain clinic one week and then six weeks later someone else would finally get to go.

Discussion

Attention needs to be paid to the educational preparation and continuous updating of staff involved in continence care provision (Rhodes and Parker, 1993; Royal College of Physicians, 1995). The current educational preparation of nurses in the ENB 978 course is inadequate for specialist nurses. A standardised specialist core module for nurses engaged in continence care should be established for delivery around the country, although it should be noted that difficulties with such modules include lack of standardisation between university departments and problems of academic credit transfer.

This chapter has aimed to systematically document the development and implementation of a new continence module. The evaluation of the programme was considered an important element of its development but could not offer a rigorous statistical evaluation due to the small numbers undertaking the module. The use of the historical control groups allowed the illustration of the CNP (experimental) group as an already interested group who were likely to be aware of and knowledgeable about continence issues and research. There was a marked difference between the groups even though they held similar grades and qualifications. This confirms that appointment of the CNP was based on a positive attitude towards research and an existing understanding of continence care.

It is likely that pre-module, greater knowledge is strongly associated with nursing grade which is linked to nursing experience. This finding has been reported elsewhere in the areas of continence (Williams *et al*, 1997) and leg ulcers (Roe *et al*, 1994). The importance of nursing experience in the provision of high quality care and development of knowledge should not be under-estimated. It is for this reason that this module linked theory and practical application so closely.

However, combining theory and practice in the module seemed to be the most problematic aspect of the programme. Access to patient clinics and sufficient patient numbers are essential to allow practical application of theoretical knowledge and can be difficult to achieve. With the current climate of evidence-based health care the module included theoretical and practical teaching on research awareness skills, including critical appraisal, enabling nurses to update their skills based on the best available evidence.

As with any education programme, student feedback on the content and delivery of the module was essential. This information was sought in a systematic way and offered useful ongoing guidance for module development. The information gained from the tape-recorded interviews supplemented the information gained from the formal educational evaluation. Perhaps future core components of an education programme on continence provision could not only be delivered by a multidisciplinary team, but also made available to a multi-disciplinary studentship as this would lead to an appreciation of roles and healthy interdisciplinary discussion.

The current Department of Health review of continence services is likely to see a prominent role for nurses in continence service provision into the next millennium (Continence Foundation, 1999). The possibility of the nurse consultant model (NHS Executive, 1998) being used in continence service provision would require clearly specified high level educational preparation.

Education programme developers rarely consider wide dissemination of details of the modules they provide locally. Ideally, educational initiatives in continence care should be reported to a recognised central multidisciplinary continence body who could disseminate information on available programmes to interested professionals. A review of post-basic education of professionals involved in continence care provision would be one way to identify what gaps exist.

This module has been shown to be effective in increasing nurses' knowledge of incontinence and can be seen as a useful model for future educational initiatives in continence care. The MRC programme focuses on community-dwelling adults aged 40 years and over and the module described targeted that group. However, additional areas of education provision for continence care providers are likely to include the following groups: residential elderly care individuals with learning disabilities, individuals requiring psychiatric care, children, women requiring maternity services, men requiring prostatic assessment and screening, and individuals with faecal incontinence.

Perhaps the preparation of good quality distance learning theory modules could be prepared by teams of 'experts' in each of these areas to link in with locally prepared practical teaching strategies.

The authors would like to thank the six CNPs originally employed on the MRC Incontinence Study: Vasanti D'Hooghe, Stephanie Duffin, Dawne Fitzsimmons, Janette Punter, Chris Rippin and Gill Wilde. The authors would also like to acknowledge the contribution of the following people who taught on and supported the module: Ms Katie Brittain, Professor Mark Castleden, Dr Francine Cheater, Professor Mike Clarke, Ms Hilary Duffin, Dr Helen Dallosso, Ms Liz Herring, Dr Jennifer Hunt, Dr Carol Jagger, Dr Aftab Laher, Dr Nelson

Lo, Mr Chris Mayne, Dr Cath McGrother, Ms Fiona Mensah, Ms Christine Norton, Mr David Osborn, Dr Sue Peet, Dr Sarah Perry, Ms Pam Robinson, Dr Tom Robinson, Ms Samantha Shaw. Particular thanks to Lesley Harris and Jennie Lucas for their administrative and clerical support. The authors would also like to thank Professor Brenda Roe for reading and commenting on an earlier manuscript.

Key points

❖ Educational initiatives in continence care should report to a recognised professional body that can disseminate information to all.

❖ Educational initiatives should offer a number of alternative delivery patterns in order to make modules more accessible, eg. distance learning.

❖ Integration of theory and practice in specialist continence modules is essential.

❖ Continence modules should draw on a multidisciplinary teaching team.

❖ Assessment of students is essential to ensure that required standards are met in both theory and practice.

❖ Initiatives to target and encourage a multidisciplinary studentship should be encouraged.

References

Brocklehurst JC (1990) Professional and public education about incontinence: the British experience. *J Am Geriatr Soc* **38**(3): 384–6

Continence Foundation (1999) Friends of the Continence Foundation. *Newsletter*. Issue three. (Available from the Continence Foundation. Tel: 020 7404 6875)

Laycock J (1995) Must do better. *Nurs Times* **91**(7): (page 5 of supplement)

NHS Executive (1998) *Nurse Consultants*. DoH, London

Perry S, Shaw C, Assassa RP *et al* (1999) An epidemiological study to establish the extent of need for health care for urinary symptoms in the community: the Leicestershire MRC incontinence study. *Proceedings of the International Continence Society* (UK) 6th Annual Meeting, 8–9 April, Edinburgh

Rhodes P, Parker G (1993) *The Role of Continence Advisers in England and Wales*. Social Policy Research Unit, University of York

Roe BH, Griffiths JM, Kenrick M, Cullum A, Hutton JL (1994) Nursing treatment of patients with chronic leg ulcers in the community. *J Clin Nurs* **3**(3): 159–68

Roe B, Wilson K, Doll H, Brooks P (1996) *An Evaluation of Health Interventions by Primary Care Teams and Continence Advisory Services on Patient Outcomes Related to Incontinence*. Report of the Health Services Research Unit. Department of Public Health and Primary Care, University of Oxford

Royal College of Physicians (1995) *Incontinence: Causes, Management and Provision of Services*. Royal College of Physicians, London

Swaffield J (1994) The management and development of continence services within the framework of the NHS and Community Care Act 1990. *J Clin Nurs* **3**(2): 119–24

UKCC (1996) *Guidelines for Professional Practice*. UKCC, London

Williams K, Crichton N, Roe B (1997) Disseminating research evidence: a controlled trial in continence care. *J Adv Nurs* **25**(4): 691–8

17

Development of a community nurse-led continence service

Noreen Shields, Cathy Thomas, Kate Benson, Kirsten Major and June Tree

Extrapolations from prevalence studies suggest that on average 56,000 adults experience urinary incontinence in Glasgow, a third of whom will have been incontinent during the last week. A review by a multidisciplinary health gain commissioning team concluded that existing continence services in Glasgow had developed opportunistically and that problems exist, eg. prescription of products without full assessment of continence problems. In response to this situation, a new community nurse-led continence service was introduced in 1995. This chapter describes the development and evaluation of this new service. For the past three years the service has employed five staff nurses and a physiotherapist. The team is solely employed to promote continence. It carries out assessments both in nursing and residential homes and community clinics. The planned evaluation will assess the effectiveness of this team in promoting continence and the future demand for continence nurse-led services.

The Department of Health's (DoH, 1991a) Agenda for Action on Continence Services estimated that between two million and three million adults in the UK experience urinary incontinence. It has been highlighted, however, that management of urinary incontinence is often inappropriate and that there is a lack of investigation of cause and an over prescription of expensive incontinence aids rather than promotion of continence (DoH, 1991b).

Failure to seek help for continence problems as a result of lack of awareness of available services or embarrassment is a major problem (Norton *et al*, 1988; Blannin, 1989). Further reports by various organisations have emphasised the potential for health gain by developing continence services that are proactive rather than reactive (Rhodes and Parker, 1993; Scottish Health Management Efficiency Group/Clinical Resource and Audit Group, 1994; Royal College of Physicians of London, 1995; Scottish Office Home and Health Department, 1995).

Norton (1997) stated that despite official support it was not clear whether all local continence services were flourishing and had a clear vision of how they should be trying to develop. In Scotland, the Scottish Health Management Efficiency Group/Clinical Resource and Audit Group report (1994) on incontinence services in the community concluded:

The problem of incontinence has been identified in a number of areas of research and possible solutions promoted in various reports. Nevertheless... in Scotland there appears to have been little progress towards achieving good management of a service which could increase quality of life for many in a cost-effective way.

A variety of health professionals are involved in continence management, eg. GPs, district nurses, health visitors, physiotherapists, social workers and voluntary service workers. However, these individuals usually have multiple roles. Traditionally, the only post dedicated solely to the promotion of continence is that of the continence adviser. However, Rhodes and Parker (1993) stated that the role of continence adviser had never been formally defined. They recommended that the continence adviser is best employed when acting in an educational and training role, with a small clinical caseload to maintain clinical expertise. Their survey of the views of continence advisers supported three models where the continence adviser's skills could be utilised to the full:

- a continence manager with one or more continence advisers
- a continence adviser/manager with a network of link or resource nurses
- a continence manager with one or more continence advisers, with a network of link or resource nurses (Rhodes and Parker, 1993).

Link nurses provide a bridge between practitioners and specialists.

The development and evaluation of such schemes has been endorsed by various professional groups involved in continence service provision (DoH, 1991a; Royal College of Physicians of London, 1995) with research indicating that nurses are well suited to developing continence promotion services (Shepherd *et al*, 1982; O'Brien *et al*, 1991; O'Brien and Long, 1995).

Link schemes have been introduced in a variety of specialties (Charalambous, 1991), particularly in hospitals. Link schemes in hospitals usually involve a nurse from each ward becoming a link person between the clinical nurse specialist and the ward. The link nurse role involves attendance at meetings where ideas and new developments can be discussed and feeding back the relevant information to nurses on the ward. This, in turn, can help improve communication with patients and their families.

Gibson (1989) described a link scheme that involved all departments in a district health authority. A member from each unit (hospital and community) was appointed to the link team to build up knowledge, expertise and resources relating to their departments' needs, with initially monthly then bimonthly meetings with the continence adviser. The continence adviser worked with link team members between meetings as needed. This scheme has not been evaluated.

This chapter describes the implementation and evaluation of a variation on the link scheme where staff act as a link between the continence advisers and ground level staff to promote good practice. In contrast, however, the Glasgow nurse-led continence team is purely community-based and is solely employed to promote continence and carry out comprehensive assessment and management programmes with individuals experiencing continence problems.

The continence service in Glasgow

In 1994, Greater Glasgow Health Board's Director of Public Health set up a multidisciplinary health gain commissioning team (HGCT) on urinary incontinence. The findings of the HGCT were that urinary incontinence is a significant problem in Glasgow (ie. 56,000 adults experience incontinence, a third of whom will have been incontinent during the previous week). The HGCT concluded that existing services had developed opportunistically without a strategic approach and that there were many associated problems (eg. high and increasing costs of products). A few models of good practice did exist, eg. the Scotland-wide, open-access, self-referral advisory continence resource centre based in the south of the city. This offers a service to sufferers and carers, both lay and professional, and has an average of 600 clinic attenders (from both within and outside Glasgow) and 3000 requests for advice per year (Dawes *et al*, 1991).

Previous research in Glasgow has illustrated that with staff dedicated to continence promotion, improvements could be gained for individuals presenting in the community and those living in nursing and residential homes (Neilson and O'Neill, 1994; McGhee *et al*, 1997).

In the context of this research, the HGCT recommended a pilot project for the extension of the community service. In reply, Greater Glasgow Health Board funded five full-time continence nurses and a half-time physiotherapist for a period of three years. An evaluation officer was also employed in line with recommendations that all innovative continence services should be subject to rigorous evaluation (Royal College of Physicians of London, 1995).

The long-term aim is to conduct a study to determine the benefits of this nurse-led continence team to the community, eg. change in problem severity (Lagro-Janssen *et al*, 1991) and social impact (Uebersax *et al*, 1995) and the costs to the NHS of continence nurses working with residents in the community and in residential/nursing home care. Different clinic models of physiotherapist/ nurse collaboration are to be examined. It is hoped that the findings of this study will aid future planning of community continence services.

Objectives of the community nurse-led continence service

In carrying out their role the community continence nurses will:

1. Assess residents in nursing/residential homes and advise on future management with the aim of improving urinary incontinence, and work closely with staff in homes to promote continence.
2. Provide assessment clinics in their locality for people who present at community clinics with urinary incontinence.
3. Act as a local information and advice resource for health professionals and carers in their locality.

The community continence physiotherapist will:

1. Provide a full physiotherapy service for urinary incontinence in one locality (ie. Clydebank/Drumchapel).
2. Educate and support continence nurses in the other four localities.
3. Carry out health promotion continence work at a family planning centre.

Role of the continence nurse

The continence nurses have a commitment to work with nursing/residential homes and in community clinics. Both these locations were chosen as evidence suggests that major continence improvements are being implemented there (Macaulay and Henry, 1990; Dawes *et al*, 1991; Neilson and O'Neill, 1994; McGhee *et al*, 1997).

Given that raising continence awareness is a major issue (Norton *et al*, 1988; Blannin, 1989), and that nurses, irrespective of grade, have been found to lack sufficient knowledge about incontinence, regarding it as 'untreatable' (Cheater, 1992), with even continence advisers demanding more training (Paterson, 1990), an important part of the continence nurse's role is to inform other professionals about continence promotion.

In relation to assessment the continence nurse follows the principles of best practice (*Table 17.1*; Norton, 1996). As well as being trained generally in the assessment and promotion of continence, nurses have more specialised skills (*Table 17.2*). The nurses see people with all types of incontinence and refer appropriately to other professionals and agencies. Examples are as follows:

- if the nurse feels that a person may benefit from anticholinergic therapy (which can help urinary frequency and bladder instability) a prescription will be requested from the GP
- if a person has no pelvic floor contraction the nurse will refer her to a physiotherapist for electrical stimulation
- if a person has suspected complications such as a second/third degree prolapse she will be referred to an urologist for urodynamic investigations.

Table 17.1. General principles of best practice in relation to continence assessment	
Type and severity of incontinence	Medical history
Current medication	Faecal voiding patterns
Mobility	Dexterity
Diet and fluid intake	Skin condition
Psychosocial factors	Environmental factors
Current product use	
Source: Norton (1996)	

Nursing assessment in nursing/residential homes

In relation to nursing and residential homes, the nurses follow the Greater Glasgow Community and Mental Health Services NHS Trust's standards of assessment and management, eg. each individual is entitled to individualised continence assessment and follow-up visits. Each nurse has a caseload of between 300 and 400 residents with continence problems.

Table 17.2: Nurses' specific skills in relation to continence promotion
Pelvic floor assessment and education of pelvic floor exercises
Bladder and habit training
Complete emptying
Intermittent self-catheterisation
Use of bladder ultrasound to detect residual urine volumes

A thorough initial assessment, including consideration of the above factors, as well as client motivation, is undertaken. In nursing and residential homes the nurses follow an initial six-month, then yearly reassessment protocol. Staff in the homes inform the continence nurse of any changes in individual residents which necessitate changes in management. A baseline assessment form was developed on the basis of previous research (Dawes *et al*, 1991), with further assessment forms developed for follow-up and reassessment visits.

Nursing assessment in community clinics

The continence nurses carry out the same comprehensive assessment in community clinics as they do in nursing/residential homes. Each nurse has approximately four clinic sessions per week. Care is individualised and the number of visits depends on the progress being made. Clients receive leaflets on the particular problem they are experiencing, eg. post micturition dribble. On average, the first visit takes 40 minutes, with follow-up visits lasting approximately 20 minutes. Clients can self-refer or be referred by any health professional, including GPs, district nurses, health visitors, family planning staff, well woman clinic staff and urology department staff.

Role of the continence physiotherapist

The physiotherapist undertakes four full physiotherapy clinic sessions per week and has a clinic at the family planning centre (FPC) once a month. The physiotherapist usually sees people with stress or urge incontinence, particularly those with poor pelvic floor muscle contraction. The service includes assessment of the pelvic floor (including vaginal examination), training in pelvic floor exercises, and interferential and biofeedback treatment if appropriate. The physiotherapist receives referrals from the FPC and explains continence promotion to clients, referring appropriately if required. Normally the client will only visit the physiotherapist once although in certain circumstances a six-month follow-up appointment is made.

    An initiative is being planned where a continence nurse and a physiotherapist, other than the continence physiotherapist, run a joint clinic. Each attender will see both clinicians unless the presenting problem is most suited to a specific professional. The continence nurse advises on bladder/habit retraining, detects residual volumes where necessary, and teaches complete emptying and intermittent self-catheterisation if appropriate. The physiotherapist assesses the pelvic floor and teaches pelvic floor muscle control, and employs interferential treatment, eg. electrical stimulation, where necessary.

Raising awareness

The continence team educates staff on the subject of continence promotion in homes and clinics, both formally and informally. The team has developed a teaching pack (overhead and hard copy) and leaflets about its service for distribution in homes and at clinics. Posters and leaflets giving details of the service and contact numbers are displayed in health centres where the team holds its clinics. In addition, general continence promotion videos are played in clinic waiting areas and generic continence promotion literature is displayed.

Role of the evaluation officer

The evaluation officer has both a monitoring and evaluation role. The monitoring role includes developing audit tools and carrying out progress reports. For example, one progress report examined the first 1317 baseline assessments carried out in nursing/residential homes. The report included details of socio-demographic characteristics, medical conditions, current medication, type and severity of incontinence experienced (Lagro-Janssen *et al*, 1991), product use and social impact of incontinence (Uebersax *et al*, 1995). It provided the focus for a discussion about the scope for promoting continence in homes.

The evaluation officer provides ongoing computer and software training to all members of the nurse-led continence team and has a facilitator role in relation to staff-management issues. One-to-one semi-structured interviews are carried out with staff at six-monthly intervals to provide feedback to both the team and managers about the process of change and innovation. The interviews cover topics such as stress, job satisfaction, support and training.

Evaluation of the community nurse-led continence service

The evaluation of the community nurse-led continence service will cover clinical, psychosocial and economic outcome measures. A random sample study of nursing/residential homes, including information on demographic characteristics, medical history, type and severity of incontinence experienced (Lagro-Janssen *et al*, 1991) and social impact (Uebersax *et al*, 1995) will be compared with control homes at baseline assessment and 12-month follow-up. In terms of economic evaluation, NHS resource use is being valued to provide a comparison between study and control homes. The economic evaluation will focus on an objective measure of change in the severity of incontinence (Lagro-Janssen *et al*, 1991). The clinical and psychosocial evaluation acknowledges that a number of other benefits will be created and that a wide range of methodologies are being employed to test for the relative importance of different attributes. In order to assess the educational output of continence nurses, level of contact and amount of advice given to staff/carers is being evaluated.

Conclusion

The community-based continence service is an innovative development. It is only by evaluating new services that the success or failure of new projects can be determined. The evaluation of this new service will aid future planning of community continence services, not only in Glasgow but also throughout the UK, and predict the likely demand for community nurse-led continence services in the future.

This study is funded by Greater Glasgow Health Board and the Community and Mental Health Service NHS Trust; however, the views expressed here are of the authors. We would like to thank all the participants in the study and the support we have had from staff in health and family planning centres, and nursing and residential homes. Special thanks go to Karen, Janey, and Les in the Continence Services Department at the Community and Mental Health NHS Trust.

Key points

❖ A total of 56,000 adults in Glasgow experience urinary incontinence, a third of whom will have been incontinent during the last week.

❖ The service in Glasgow has tended to manage incontinence rather than promote continence.

❖ A three-year study is being carried out to assess the effectiveness of five staff nurses and a half-time physiotherapist solely promoting continence in nursing/residential homes and community clinics.

❖ The evaluation of the community nurse-led continence service is considering clinical, psychosocial and economic outcome measures.

❖ The study should provide information that is relevant to the planning of continence services in Glasgow and throughout the UK.

References

Blannin JP (1989) The sooner the better! Teaching continence promotion to women. *Prof Nurse* **5**(3): 149–52

Charalambous L (1991) Development of the link nurse role in clinical settings. *Nurs Times* **11**(91): 36–7

Cheater FM (1992) Nurses' educational preparation and knowledge concerning continence promotion. *J Adv Nurs* **17**: 328–38

Dawes H, Cherry L, Ballentyne M *et al* (1991) Advice for all. *Nurs Times* **87**(44): 56–62

DoH (1991a) *An Agenda for Action on Continence Services.* Community Services Division, Department of Health, London

DoH (1991b) *NHS Management Letter* (91)28. Department of Health, London

Gibson E (1989) Coordinating continence care. *Nurs Times* **85**(7): 73–5

Lagro-Janssen ALM, Smits AJA, van Weel C (1991) Women with urinary incontinence — self-perceived worries and general practitioners' knowledge of the problems. *Br J Gen Practice* **40**: 331–4

McGhee·M, O'Neill K, Major K *et al* (1997) Evaluation of a nurse-led continence service in the South West of Glasgow. *J Adv Nurs* **26**: 723–8

Macauley M, Henry G (1990) Drop in and do well. *Nurs Times* **86**(46): 65–6

Neilson A, O'Neill KF (1994) *Community-Based Audit of Continence in Over Seventy Fives.* Report to Medical Audit Committee, Glasgow

Norton C (1996) *Nursing for Continence.* 2nd edn. Beaconsfield Publishers, Beaconsfield

Norton C (1997) Providing appropriate continence services: an overview. *Nurs Standard* **10**(40): 41–5

Norton PA, MacDonald LD, Sedgwick PM *et al* (1988) Distress and delay associated with urinary incontinence, frequency and urgency in women. *Br Med J* **297**: 1187–9

O'Brien J, Austin M, Sethi P *et al* (1991) Urinary incontinence: prevalence, need for treatment and effectiveness by nurses. *Br Med J* **303**: 1308–12

O'Brien J, Long H (1995) Urinary incontinence: long-term effectiveness of nursing intervention in primary care. *Br Med J* **311**: 1208

Paterson H (1990) Education wanted. *Nurs Times* **86**(22): 71

Royal College of Physicians of London (1995) *Incontinence: Causes, Management and Provision of Services.* Royal College of Physicians, London

Rhodes P, Parker G (1993) *The Role of Continence Advisers in England and Wales.* Social Policy and Research Unit, University of York

Scottish Health Management Efficiency Group/Clinical Resource and Audit Group (1994) *SCOTMEG Project 41.* Incontinence Services in the Community, Trinity Park House, Edinburgh

Scottish Office Home and Health Department (1995) *A Research Agenda for the Effective Recognition and Management of Urinary and Faecal Incontinence.* SOHHD, Edinburgh

Shepherd AM, Blannin JP, Feneley RCL (1982) Changing attitudes in the management of urinary incontinence — the need for specialist nursing. *Br Med J* **284**: 645–6

Uebersax JS, Wyman JF, Shumaker SA *et al* (1995) Short forms to assess life quality symptom distress in women: the incontinence impact questionnaire and urogenital distress inventory. *Neurol Urodyn* **14**: 131–9

18
Pathways for continence care: background and audit

Valerie Bayliss, Maggie Cherry, Rachel Locke and Liz Salter

Trusts in Basingstoke, Swindon and Salisbury have collaborated in supporting their continence advisers in moving from finance-driven assessment data to evidence-based care pathways and the provision of patient information. This chapter identifies the background and approach to care pathways and addresses the quality issues. It details the issues facing continence advisers and how care pathways may help to address them. Furthermore, it describes a baseline audit which was carried out to ensure that facts rather than beliefs were being used and this demonstrated that little advice or treatment was actually reaching the patient.

Care pathways map out a timed process of patient-focused care which specifies key events, tests and assessments to produce the best prescribed outcomes, within the limits of the resources available, for an appropriate episode of care (Wilson, 1992). In practice, this process seeks to describe in advance the care of patients within specific case types. These may include diagnosis (eg. myocardial infarction), procedure (endoscopy) or condition (pain).

Within the specific case type there are common strands (ie. blood pressure for myocardial infarction, sedation for endoscopy, response to analgesia for pain) which are mapped out on the pathway and which are then used as a guideline for the practitioner. The practitioner uses his/her clinical judgement to decide whether to follow the care on the pathway or to deviate from it. Such deviations are recorded as part of the pathway documentation, thus providing the means by which care may be individualised (Johnson, 1997).

Such deviations are known as variances. Interventions may have much in common, but patients are different and the skill of the practitioner is in adapting interventions to the individual patient. Care pathways are useful because of their great potential for enhancing the quality of care and the overall picture which they can give of the patient's condition (Walsh, 1998).

Background

Continence advisers, like many other nurses, have problems in ensuring that services to patients within their specialty provide equitable evidence-based care. Efficiency and quality should go hand in hand as both are essential to fairness. Patients suffer if resources are not used to their best effect just as they suffer if quality varies (Department of Health, 1997). Incontinence is becoming recognised as a common condition which can be easily cured or better managed (Getliffe and Dolman, 1997). Many trusts employ continence advisers to provide a direct service to patients and education is considered to be one of the most important aspects of that role (Rhodes and Parker, 1993).

It has long been recognised that good quality assessment will define problems and a knowledgeable practitioner will be able to suggest solutions. Studies have shown a 70–80% cure or improvement rate in primary care by enthusiasts (Royal College of Physicians, 1995). Indeed, the Charter for Continence (Continence Foundation, 1995) states that the individual has the right to full continence assessment. To this end, most continence advisers have designed assessment forms for trust-wide use as a way of collecting data and have provided in-service training for other healthcare professionals. Part of the training process is to provide education in order that healthcare professionals can promote good continence care.

Education can help to provide high quality nursing care, thus reducing the need for continence pads and saving money. Many continence advisers have been appointed in the expectation that they will be able to effect a reduction in expenditure by reducing patients' reliance on incontinence products (Rhodes and Parker, 1993).

Conflicts and priorities

Most continence advisers have responsibility for the budgetary control of continence aids. Many are poorly funded and have to apply cost controls. This has caused a shortage in some continence services, some of which have to wait for products due to a lack of funding (Dolman, 1998).

There is also an issue regarding cost *vs* quality. The boundaries between the quality of continence care and budgetary control have become blurred as many continence advisers have instituted policies which require a continence assessment form to be completed before a continence pad can be used. Moreover, the importance of quality, equity and standards are emphasised throughout *A First Class Service* (DoH, 1998).

However, healthcare professionals have many demands on their time. Increasing levels of dependence in the community mean that community nurses must prioritise their caseloads and a continence assessment has low priority against, for example, meeting the needs of a terminally ill patient. Not all nurses are particularly motivated by continence issues or view them as a great priority. This must be seen against the background of the health needs of a nurse's whole caseload and should not be regarded as a criticism of individual practitioners, simply a statement of reality.

To facilitate better levels of continence care, continence advisers provide ongoing training and education. However, in practice, it is the same interested nurses who regularly attend the education sessions, thus the motivation of the individual nurse can determine the quality of the service provided.

The objective of trying to reduce spending on continence products has resulted in assessment becoming a way of controlling costs rather than providing high quality care to the incontinent person. The authors found that when continence assessment takes place by healthcare professionals other than continence advisers it is with the aim of providing a pad. Indeed, it is not uncommon for the assessment to be referred to as a pad assessment rather than a continence assessment.

Assessment forms are submitted to the continence adviser for checking for quality issues and because of the need for cost-containment. For example, some trusts have a policy of supplying no more that four pads per 24-hour period. This checking of the assessment forms can cause conflict between continence advisers and other healthcare professionals to the detriment of the patient. This practice is strongly discouraged in *Good Practice in Continence Services* (2000).

The beginning of the project

The authors met informally and discovered that the situation described above was common to all of them. After further discussion they identified the issues shown in *Table 18.1*.

Table 18.1: Common issues facing continence advisers
No consistency of practice within trusts
Clinical assessment driven by financial constraint
Lack of interest in continence issues from nurses in general
Continence issues not a priority for many healthcare professionals
Wasting of clinical specialists' time — checking paperwork, dealing with inappropriate referrals
Little use of new research by continence advisers and nurses in general
Poor delivery of care in community and primary care

Baseline audit

The first step in the process was to check that these beliefs were grounded in fact. To this end a baseline audit was undertaken of 100 patients in each of the three trusts. A postal questionnaire was sent to randomly selected community patients who had recently (within the last six months) been assessed by a community nurse. Each of the authors had, over a period of time, undertaken regular education and training sessions with the community staff concerned. However, for the purposes of eliminating bias, the audit, and the audit analysis, were carried out by the Audit Department at Odstock Hospital, Salisbury.

Of the patients, 97% had their assessment carried out by a district nurse; 83% were female and 90% were over the age of 60. Although urine testing should have formed part of the assessment only 4% had provided a sample at their initial assessment. Only 14% had a catheter passed to check for residual urine, although this too should have formed part of the assessment (the authors suspect that a lack of interest in continence care and a belief that the patient would end up with pads anyway made for cursory continence assessment).

Patients were asked a series of questions including:

- what advice they had been given
- what tests they had received
- what the long-term view of their prognosis was
- their levels of incontinence.

Patients were also asked about their current continence status (*Table 18.2*) since their discussion with the nurse. A high response rate was not expected as it was felt that patients may be too embarrassed to complete the question- naires despite the assurances of anonymity. A response rate of 30–40% is usually expected from postal questionnaires (McNeill, 1990). However, despite low expectations the response rate was between 65% and 69% which showed that this particular group of incontinent patients wanted to be involved in their care. Furthermore, many of the questionnaires were written in detail, demonstrating that the patients wanted to share their feelings and perceptions. It is interesting to note that the majority of the comments were concerned with aspects of treatment not provision or quality of products.

Table 18.2: How would you describe your incontinence problem?	
My incontinence has become worse	22%
My incontinence has remained about the same	55%
My incontinence has improved slightly	14%
My incontinence has improved greatly	6%
Incontinence is no longer a problem for me	2%
No data	2%

At the same time an audit of the patients' assessment forms was undertaken to see how closely the information provided by the community nurses matched the patients' understanding (the community nurses also wrote their comments on the assessment forms) (*Table 18.3*). The purpose of this was to study the patients' perceptions of the care that they had received. For example, 27% of community nurses stated on the assessment forms that they had taught pelvic floor exercises, but only 7% of patients remembered being taught them. This did not necessarily demonstrate that patients had not been taught pelvic floor exercises but the fact that they did not remember them illustrated a need for better patient information.

The results from each trust were broadly similar and are therefore combined. The results reinforced the belief that patients did not receive either an equitable service or appropriate information. The majority of patients were motivated enough to complete the questionnaire and many stated that they wished to improve their continence status. It is not suggested that any patients' continence status worsened as a result of nursing intervention, but rather that more of the care could have been improved.

Table 18.3: Action taken as described in assessment form	
Action taken	**% of patients**
Patient given pads	100
Patient educated about pelvic floor exercises	27
Patient given bladder training	10
Patient given advice on fluids	8
Patient given advice on mobility	7
Patient referred to other healthcare professional	7
Patient given urine test	4
Patient's medication reviewed	4
Patient given dietary advice	4
Patient's frequency/volume of micturition charted	3

Only 20% of the patients showed some improvement, a figure markedly below that given by the Royal College of Physicians, ie. 70–80%. There was, indeed, evidence to show that the delivery of continence care in the community could be improved.

The authors then identified a list of aims for quality continence services (*Table 18.4*). This was then turned into a list of how the service could be improved, both for staff and patients.

Table 18.4: Aims for quality continence services
Patient focused
Use evidence-based practice or agreed best practice where evidence base is not available
Separate clinical element from budgetary control
Deliver consistency of care wherever and to whoever the patient presents
No duplication of clinical tests, information or administration
Flexible assessment tools should be provided by continence advisers for both healthcare professionals and patients
Healthcare professionals should be accountable for the provision of care which should be given in partnership with patients
Care must be practical, auditable, transferable and user friendly
Care should be provided within existing resources

The solution that seemed to meet all the objectives was the care pathway process which anticipates and describes, in advance, the care of patients within specific case types. Moreover, regular monitoring and review change the pathway as advances are made and variances are identified. The pathway would provide the appropriate intervention(s) while allowing clinical freedom through the variance-tracking process.

As a result of the audit, each trust was approached with a proposal asking for both the time and resources to undertake further development. The continence advisers were granted study leave and the Salisbury Healthcare NHS Trust and Loddon NHS Trust further supported the project by donating £2000 each.

Creating an evidence base

The authors contacted various trusts who were already some way into instituting the care pathway process and also spoke to the care pathway coordinator at Salisbury Healthcare NHS Trust who gave valuable advice and help. However, no other trust could be found which had tried to adapt the care pathway process for use with continence problems. As no evidence could be traced of full continence care pathways, the authors decided to opt for developing a research-based process which means that no item can appear anywhere (pathways or patient information) without research to support it.

As nurses become more accountable for the care they provide it is important that care is based on the best clinical practice and systemic reviews of research findings (RCN, 1996). Accessing and appraising evidence is rapidly becoming a core clinical competency and clinical decisions can no longer be based on opinion alone (Scally and Donaldson, 1998). To this end, funding was used to employ a postdoctoral research assistant as expert help was needed in identifying the type and quality of the research. Guidance was also sought from an independent care pathways consultant.

The authors agreed that the care pathway would be directed at healthcare professionals who had general skills but not necessarily any specialist knowledge. Thus, a general nurse would need no specialist skills in the field of continence care as all the basic steps in assessment, treatment and action would be set out in the pathway. This was to try to neutralise inequalities in knowledge levels and make research-based continence care available to all patients.

An enormous amount of work has been undertaken by the project team in order to bring it to fruition. The results of the baseline audit were clear in that prescribed education was not particularly effective in reaching the patient, although it may reach the nurse. The aim became to use the nurse as a skilled conductor to get quality, evidence-based information to the patient.

Key points

❖ Specialist nurses need to address the quality issues set out by the Government and Department of Health.

❖ The quality of continence assessment is confused by financial constraint.

❖ Advice and treatment for improving continence status is not reaching the patient.

❖ Care pathways provide for an equitable minimum standard of service for all.

❖ Expert scientific validation ensures that evidence-based practice translates from theory into reality.

References

Continence Foundation (1995) *Charter for Continence.* Continence Foundation, London

Dolman (1998) Strategies to promote continence in the community. *Br J Comm Nurs* **33**(8): 385–392

DoH (1997) *The New NHS — modern, dependable.* HMSO London

DoH (1998) *A First Class Service — Quality in the New NHS.* HMSO, London

DoH (2000) *Good Practice in Continence Services.* Department of Health, London

Getliffe K, Dolman M (1997) *Promoting Continence.* Ballière Tindall, London

Johnson S (1997) *Pathways of Care.* Blackwell Science, Oxford

McNeill P (1990) *Research Methods.* Routledge, London

Rhodes P, Parker G (1993) *The Role of Continence Advisers in England and Wales Social Policy.* Research Unit, University of York

RCN (1996) *Clinical Effectiveness.* Royal College of Nursing, London

Royal College of Physicians (1995) *Incontinence — Causes, Management and Provision of Services.* Royal College of Physicians, London

Scally G, Donaldson LJ (1998) Clinical governance and the drive for quality improvement in the new NHS in England. *Br Med J* **317**: 61–5

Walsh M (1998) *Models and Critical Pathways in Clinical Nursing.* Ballière Tindall, London

Wilson J (1992) *An Introduction to Multidisciplinary Pathways of Care.* Northern Region Health Authority, Newcastle upon Tyne

19

Male catheterisation by female nurses: a small-scale survey

Gary Porter-Jones

A small-scale questionnaire survey of nurses in one Welsh district general hospital examined the views of nurses in relation to catheterisation of male patients. The findings demonstrate that while most nurses agree that it is acceptable for females to catheterise male patients, most female nurses do not undertake the procedure as they incorrectly believe that there are either local or national policies that prevent patients from being catheterised by nurses of the opposite sex. This often results in patients waiting longer than necessary to be catheterised, and nurses (usually male nurses) from other clinical areas being requested to catheterise a patient for whom they are not caring. Such beliefs and practices stifle the development of knowledge on this issue.

The nursing literature contains an abundance of studies on catheters and the care of catheters (Rigby, 1998; Winn, 1998). This is not surprising given the enormous numbers of catheters in use in hospitals (10% of inpatients is the figure widely quoted) (Mulhall *et al*, 1988; Falkiner, 1993; Winson, 1997) and in the community (an estimated 4% of patients receiving nursing care have a catheter) (Getliffe and Mulhall, 1991), and the numerous situations where catheterisation may be indicated (*Table 19.1*). Such studies are essential in order that we may constantly question our practice and ensure that it is based in evidence. Examining a widespread phenomenon can only be beneficial to the development of the nursing profession.

One aspect of catheterisation that generates controversy is the notion of patients being catheterised by persons of the opposite sex. This chapter focuses on the catheterisation of male patients by female nurses.

Although this issue is potentially controversial, there have been relatively few studies on it, despite it being an issue that affects practice not only locally but also nationally. This problem was identified by Fader (1986) at a time when many districts would not allow female nurses to catheterise

Table 19.1: Situations necessitating catheterisation
Relief of acute or chronic retention of urine
Determination of residual urine volume
Accurate measurement of urine output
Emptying of the bladder pre-, peri- and postoperatively
Bladder irrigation
Introduction of drugs into the bladder
Performance of bladder function tests
To bypass obstruction

male patients. The rationale underlying this stance was questioned and it was argued that this policy should be changed in order that patients might benefit. Pomfret (1993) also found that many females were not catheterising male patients, although by this time there was often no policy preventing this practice; tradition appeared to be the barrier to change in many cases.

Also, many will recognise the paradoxical situation of a female nurse calling out a female doctor to catheterise a male patient or change the catheter. Despite being noted over 20 years ago (Nelson, 1978), such practice is often still in evidence today. This would appear to be one area of nursing practice that has failed to develop.

In congruence with these findings, the author noted that many female nurses in his place of work do not catheterise male patients. Female nurses frequently refuse to undertake this procedure, and thereby often cause the patient unnecessary and prolonged discomfort. Also, as the only male member of the qualified nursing staff within the department of urology, the author was frequently requested to visit other wards within the hospital, purely to catheterise a male patient. It would not be unusual to receive two or more of these requests in one day. This highlights three factors that give cause for concern:

- in most circumstances it would be inconvenient, and often impossible, to do this owing to demands on the ward
- there are potential risks in undertaking catheterisation without knowledge of the patient's medical history and, most importantly, urinary tract history
- the practice is unnecessary.

Aim of the study

The author decided to examine this issue more closely to identify the reasons for this practice. With this knowledge he hoped to be able to develop a mechanism for overcoming this issue. All things considered, this practice is unnecessary and inconveniences both the patient and the person undertaking the procedure.

Method

Pilot

As a form of pilot study, some of the issues surrounding catheterisation by a person of the opposite sex were discussed with a number of nurses who constituted the study population (ie. qualified nurses working in the hospital in which the study took place). This exercise identified three issues that needed to be addressed (*Table 19.2*) and thus gave direction to the questionnaire.

Table 19.2: Main themes emerging from discussions with qualified nurses
1. Uncertainty about local policy relating to the issue of nurses catheterising patients of the opposite sex.
2. Unfamiliarity with the procedure of male catheterisation.
3. The belief that a patient should be catheterised by a person of the same sex.

In order to address the issue of policy, discussion was held with hospital senior nurse managers, including the Executive Nurse Director with whom it was clarified that there was no local policy preventing nurses from catheterising patients of the opposite sex purely on gender grounds. The UKCC's stance was similar, while reinforcing that, through an individual's accountability, professional competence and patients' wishes are the factors that should determine professional practice (UKCC, personal communication).

Questionnaire

The questionnaire was developed using the information gained in the pilot study. It focused on four main factors addressing the relevant issues related to the notion of female nurses catheterising male patients (*Table 19.3*). The questionnaire was distributed to both male and female nurses in order to obtain as valuable qualitative data as possible. Quantification of data was restricted to rudimentary counting, expressing the findings as percentages of responses. The questionnaire, with full instructions, was sent to 83 qualified nurses (both first and second level) on six wards within the hospital: two surgical wards, two medical wards and two orthopaedic wards. An addressed return envelope was included to promote a satisfactory response rate. The hospital internal mail system was used for returns.

Table 19.3: Content of the questionnaire
What are your thoughts about female nurses catheterising male patients?
As far as you know, what is the Gwynedd Hospitals NHS Trust's policy on this issue?
Have you ever catheterised a male patient? If 'yes', how did you learn about the procedure?
If 'yes', do you feel competent in carrying this out?
If 'no', are there any special reasons for this?
What are your thoughts about an in-service education programme aimed at developing knowledge about the procedure?
Please feel free to add any comments you think are important

Sample

The sample for this study was purposively selected and included all qualified nurses on the above mentioned wards. It is considered that the sample size and method of selection are such that generalisability to the study population as a whole is reasonable, while recognising that purposive sampling methods offer a poor foundation for generalisability on a wider plane.

Equally important are the advantages of such a technique, ie. economy and convenience — extremely pertinent issues in such a small-scale study. Generalisability was not an aim of this study; rather, an approach was adopted that demonstrated concern for individual situations that can be deliberately explored in isolation (Hockey, 1991).

Reliability and validity

The evaluation of reliability and validity within this study stems from the methods described by Glaser and Strauss (1967), in which the findings were returned to the original respondents from whom the data were obtained. The data were examined by the nurses who formed the initial pilot group. In addition, the researcher's interpretation of responses was clarified by the individual who gave that response. In all cases the respondents agreed that their responses had been correctly interpreted. This method was undertaken with 51% (31 nurses) of the sample. The original respondents offered feedback that was used to establish both reliability and validity.

Data analysis

Analysis of data was relatively straightforward. The content of the questionnaire formed categories into which responses were placed. The terminology used in the questionnaire was such that responses clearly fell into positive or negative categories, with only the 5% expressing uncertainty falling into neither category. These data were then totalled and expressed as percentages of the overall response.

Results

A total of 61 completed questionnaires were returned, giving a 73% response rate.

Eighty-five per cent of respondents (52 nurses) agreed that it was acceptable for female nurses to catheterise male patients, 10% (six nurses) did not feel it was acceptable, and 5% (three nurses) were uncertain.

Only 7% (four nurses) had ever catheterised a male patient, and all of these felt competent in doing so.

Ninety per cent (55 nurses) incorrectly believed that a policy exists which prevents female nurses from catheterising male patients; only 7% (four nurses) correctly indicated that no policy exists; and 3% (two nurses) were unsure about any policies.

An in-service education package aimed at developing knowledge about the subject was considered a good idea by 97% (59 nurses), while the remaining 3% (two nurses) did not seem to understand the question.

Discussion

Although the majority of respondents (85%) supported the notion of female nurses catheterising male patients (*Figure 19.1*), very few (7%) had ever undertaken the procedure. An extremely high proportion (93%) were not aware that it is permissible for a female nurse to catheterise a male patient (*Figure 19.2*). The vast majority believe that policies, either local or central, prevent this from taking place. This may be a major reason for the failure in development of knowledge and attitudes.

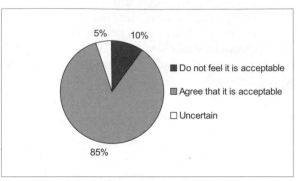

Figure 19.1: Respondents' thoughts about female nurses catheterising male patients

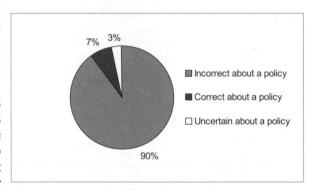

Of the six nurses (10%) who thought it was not acceptable for men to be catheterised by women, two commented that they thought a male patient would prefer to be catheterised by a male member of staff as it is too intimate a procedure for people of the opposite sex to undertake.

Figure 19.2: Respondents' knowledge of their hospital's policy on female nurses catheterising male patients

The remaining four nurses expressed a view that could be considered to stem from tradition, commenting that:

> *Men have always been catheterised by men in the past and this has never been questioned.*

and,

> *This issue has never been seen as a problem before so why should it do so now?*

It is noteworthy that whereas the comment by the first two nurses is based on what might be considered valid reasoning, and reflects a genuine concern for the interests of the patient, the last two appear to be based merely on a traditionalist perspective, and therefore form a poor foundation for argument. Such attitudes do little to promote the evidence base that should underpin the nursing profession.

Interestingly, the 7% (four nurses) who correctly indicated that no policy exists were the same four nurses who had catheterised male patients. This is encouraging as it supports the notion that acquiring knowledge can lead to a change in practice.

Local policy and/or guidelines do not address the issue of gender in relation to catheterisation. Therefore, from a policy perspective, it is quite acceptable for a female to catheterise a male and a male to catheterise a female. Possibly the tenacity with which the nursing profession has held onto traditional practices (Hicks, 1997; Walshe *et al*, 1995) has prevented this from taking place in the past. The nursing profession has relied a great deal on tradition for guiding its future, whereas experience demonstrates that evidence-based practice is by far a better tool with which to extend the boundaries of our profession.

Although neither local policy nor governing body offers guidance on gender issues, the UKCC is quite explicit in pointing out to nurses that they must acknowledge limitations to their competence and that these must not be exceeded (UKCC, 1992). Nurses are reminded that, as accountable individuals, they are responsible for attaining and developing their competence in undertaking any procedure and this holds true for catheterisation. With certification now increasingly becoming a thing of the past, individual nurses are also responsible for deciding when they become competent.

One of the most important factors in relation to the catheterisation of patients is that the wishes of the patient are paramount and should be respected at all times, where possible. If a male patient makes it clear that he would prefer a male member of staff to insert his catheter, this should be respected and every attempt should be made to carry out his wishes. The same would obviously apply with female patients.

It is interesting that the notion of male nurses catheterising female patients does not generate the same level of controversy. Perhaps this is due to the preponderance of female nurses, which prevents this from becoming an issue at the outset. If a female patient needs catheterising, it is highly likely that there will be a female member of staff available to do this.

Discussion with student nurses also revealed that they were informed, as part of their nurse education, that insertion of catheters by a person of the opposite sex was not allowed. Furthermore, the few who questioned why this was so were informed that local policy prevented this practice. This was also the experience of students questioned from various other nurse education establishments nationally, suggesting that it is a more widespread issue than this study suggests. Although not incorporated into this study, as it was only identified after its completion, it is an interesting finding that warrants further investigation.

Woollons (1996) also reports a lack of knowledge necessary to ensure optimal care of catheterised patients, and suggests that inadequate emphasis on the use of catheters by educationalists may account for this. It would therefore appear that newly qualified nurses are entering clinical practice misinformed, and perpetuating the situation.

Conclusion

This small-scale survey demonstrates that the issue of catheterising patients is controversial at times. The level of knowledge about gender issues relating to the subject appears to be deficient and it is likely that negative attitudes will persist and prevent the continuance and development of evidence-based practice. It is essential that the root of this misinformation is identified and targeted for change. Only when this has been established can attitudes, and ultimately practice, begin to evolve.

Gender is not an issue that prevents a practitioner from catheterising a patient, but the absence of professional competence and the wishes of the patient are such issues. The former must be identified and never exceeded and the latter must be respected whenever possible.

Once nurses are aware that they are able to undertake this procedure, it is essential that they are reminded of the specifications of the UKCC in relation to attaining, developing and recognising and maintaining competence. Those eager to develop knowledge and skills in this field should be given the opportunity to do so through structured educational programmes.

There may be local policies elsewhere that dictate who is, or is not, permitted to perform this procedure, but it is neither local policy at the hospital in which this study was undertaken, nor the policy of the UKCC, despite what many nurses may believe. It is time, however, that the nursing profession addresses this issue, either centrally or through locally developed initiatives, in order that patients receive catheter care of the highest quality, regardless of the gender of their nurse.

Recommendations

Now that the ambiguity surrounding male catheterisation, which has existed for so long, has been identified, health authorities and hospitals should make clear their stance on gender issues in relation to catheterisation so that the situation is clarified locally. It is essential that their approach is non-gender biased. The development of nursing in this area relies on this.

Educational initiatives should be implemented to redress the deficit in present knowledge on this subject and adequately prepare nurses for undertaking the procedure. With the vast majority (97%) of nurses in this study supporting the idea of an educational programme, it would be unfair and possibly unethical to ignore their enthusiasm by doing nothing further locally. The author, therefore, has developed such a learning tool in conjunction with expert nursing and medical practitioners and senior educationalists, the aim of which is to meet the needs of these people in theoretical and practical terms and eventually change common practices.

It is essential that student nurses be correctly informed of any local policies pertaining to catheterisation, and of the position of the UKCC on this issue. The identification of misinformation in this area suggests that further study should be undertaken with a student nurse focus. As they are the nurses of the future, it is imperative that they begin their careers with a sound knowledge base. A copy of this study will be forwarded to the relevant local educational establishments.

Further investigation to identify and address issues lying beyond the parameters of this small scale study is warranted.

Key points

❖ Men requiring catheterisation in hospital is a common occurrence.

❖ Many female nurses do not undertake this procedure as they incorrectly believe that they are not permitted to do so because of local or national policy.

❖ Many student nurses complete their training, having been incorrectly informed about gender issues and male catheterisation. This reflects the need for evidence-based practice as opposed to practice stemming from tradition.

❖ The patient's wishes are paramount and should be respected whenever possible.

References

Fader M (1986) Continence: new thoughts on male catheterisation. *Nurs Times* **82**(15): 64–6
Falkiner FR (1993) The insertion and management of indwelling urethral catheters: minimising the risk of infection. *J Hosp Infect* **25**: 79–90
Getliffe KA, Mulhall AB (1991) The encrustation of indwelling catheters. *Br J Urol* **67**: 337–41
Glaser BG, Strauss AL (1967) *The Discovery of Grounded Theory. Strategies for Qualitative Research*. Aldine, Chicago
Hicks C (1997) The dilemma of incorporating research into clinical practice. *Br J Nurs* **6**: 511–15
Hockey L (1991) The nature and purpose of research. In: Cormack D, ed. *The Research Process in Nursing*. 2nd edn. Blackwell Scientific, London
Mulhall AB, Chapman RG, Crow RA (1988) Catheters: the acquisition of bacteriuria; emptying urinary drainage bags; meatal cleansing. *Nurs Times* **84**(4): 61–9
Nelson J (1978) Forbidden thoughts. *Nurs Times* **74**(42): 17–21
Pomfret I (1993) Catheters: men only. *Nurs Times* **89**(8): 55–8
Rigby D (1998) Long-term catheter care. *Prof Nurse* **13**(5): s14–s15
UKCC (1992) *Code of Professional Conduct for the Nurse, Midwife and Health Visitor*. Paragraph 2, Clause 4. UKCC, London
Walshe K, Ham C, Appleby J (1995) Given in evidence. *Health Serv J* **105**: 28–9
Winn C (1998) Complications with urinary catheters. *Prof Nurse* **13**(5): s7–s10
Winson L (1997) Catheterisation: a need for improved patient management. *Br J Nurs* **6**: 1229–52
Woollons S (1996) Urinary catheters for long-term use. *Prof Nurse* **11**: 825–32

20

Implementing evidence-based practice for urinary catheterisation

Freya Adams and Mary Cooke

Nursing development units (NDUs) are ideal centres for the critical examination of clinical nursing practice. In addition, staff are enabled to clarify appropriate and effective methods of care and interventions based on evidence to date (Department of Health, 1993, 1998; English National Board [ENB], 1996, 1997; Centre for Policy in Nursing Research, 1997). In July 1996, the staff within the cardiology NDU at Addenbrooke's NHS Trust looked at the potential for various projects that were central to practice. One concerned the management of urinary catheters. A pilot study was initiated, one outcome of which was the design of a project checklist based on Sackett *et al*'s definition of evidence-based practice (EBP) (Sackett *et al*, 1997). In this chapter, the aims and intentions of the project are evaluated in relation to the problems associated with implementing evidence. In addition, the framework of the White Paper (DoH, 1998) is examined against the need for an organisational infrastructure, which is required to enable achievement of the outcomes of EBP. The benefits of the project are outlined, both in the changes to practice and for the unit. Recommendations for other professionals are also offered, as there are few recorded experiences in the literature of implementation of EBP, the process framework required and the costs involved.

Sackett *et al* (1997) view evidence-based practice (EBP) as comprising the following stages:

- identifying a problem
- finding an answer through literature searches and critiques
- implementing the change
- evaluating the change.

EBP can therefore be seen as any research or evidence, eg. clinician experience and manufacturers' recommendations, that can be applied in practice to benefit health care in terms of patients' psychological, physical and social well-being, and cost-effectiveness.

Rationale for project

Clinical nursing staff in the cardiology nursing development unit (NDU) at

Addenbrooke's NHS Trust Hospital decided to design a pilot project for the implementation of EBP in relation to the management of short-term urinary catheters. The primary aims and objectives of this project were:

- to design guidelines for staff in the NDU on the management of short-term indwelling urinary catheters
- to promote and set the standard and therefore the consistency of care based on evidence.

The secondary aims and objectives were:

- to experience the process of implementing EBP
- to develop a method of learning that has a defined outcome
- to identify and resolve problems with a clinically focused and patient-centred activity
- to disseminate the outcomes to trust staff and make recommendations for the future.

Short-term urinary catheters are defined as catheters that are *in situ* for less than 28 days (Bard, 1997). Cardiology patients often need to be catheterised so that their urinary output and the ability of the cardiac muscle to regain haemodynamic stability can be monitored (Marieb, 1996). Urethral catheterisation and its management is therefore an essential nursing activity within the cardiology unit. On investigation there were no local written guidelines or trust policies for staff concerning urethral catheterisation, and observation showed that there was little evidence of consistent practice. As Sackett *et al* (1997) state, the identification of this problem is the initial stage in the process of introducing EBP. A working party of staff was formed to determine the completion of the identified project and an F grade sister emerged as the project's leader.

Stages of the project

Table 20.1 lists the various stages of the project. The second stage 'Assessment' involved obtaining information to support and sustain the programme, beginning with carrying out a literature search and critical analysis, and seeking expert advice from consultant urologists, regional continence advisers and the nursing research adviser. Project objectives were formed through auditing current practice. Lewin's (1951) process of 'force field analysis' was applied in order to identify the driving and restraining forces of the work, together with identifying any individuals who were committed to support and help with the project (*Figure 20.1*).

An exhaustive literature review from the last 10 years using CINAHL and Cochrane databases was completed using the search words 'urinary catheters', 'catheters' and 'indwelling catheters'. This resulted in the collection of 45 relevant and appropriate articles. Manufacturers' information was collated separately from industrial sources and representatives.

Table 20.1: Stages of the project		
Stage	**Action**	**Date of completion**
1. Identify problem	Identify working group and leader	January 1997
2. Assessment	Obtain information Critique literature Make contact with experts Form project objectives	April 1997
3. Analyse situation	Commitment planning Force field analysis Review current practice	April 1997
4. Planning	Project strategy and time frames Communication strategy	June 1997
5. Implementation	Implement planning phase strategy Monitor and control	August 1997
6. Evaluation	Implement evaluation strategy Assess change in practice	December, 1999
7. Dissemination of information	Feedback to appropriate staff members and groups within the trust Recommendations for future	December, 1999

Driving forces	**Equilibrium**	**Restraining forces**
Project leader and working party		Time constraints: Individual time-out Group meetings
Unit manager support		Financial implications
Staff motivation within NDU		Reduced establishments
Research given high priority		Stress associated with increase workload
Excellent resources: Expertise Library Database		Lack of knowledge and experience

Figure 20.1: The driving and restraining forces of the project.
Adapted from Lewin's (1951) 'force field analysis'

The project working party then began to examine methods of educating the ward staff to keep them informed of the project stages and to share the process. The most effective way of doing this was seen to be through:

- disseminating the findings of the literature review, eg. through posters and teaching sessions
- improving management of care by developing written and agreed guidelines for staff based on evidence

Derby Hospital NHS
Foundation Trust
01332 788146

Mail: dhft.library@nhs.net

Self Service Receipt for Borrowing

Patron: Mrs Agnes Nakigudde

Title: Management of continence and urinary cath
Item: T10600
Due Back: 16/07/2015

Title: Nursing for continence.
Item: 100327086X
Due Back: 16/07/2015

Total Borrowing: 2
21/05/2015 11.19 54

Thank you and see you soon

- documenting all episodes of urinary catheterisation using a designated documentation form.

The NDU is now working through the implementation stage of the project. The working party is collectively responsible for ensuring that changes in practice are occurring. Quarterly meetings consist of progress reports and feedback, where problems encountered are discerned and solutions are determined.

One of the difficulties was found to be how to disseminate to other nurses in the trust the findings from the literature review and the application of the criteria to define the specific use of catheters, their insertion and *in situ* care. At this stage it became clear that there was no framework in the trust for dissemination, or strategies to support the implementation of EBP. The senior nurse director was engaged to plan presentations to ward staff, senior staff and managers. In addition, presentations have been undertaken at two international nursing conferences.

The EBP working party group aims to assess progress within the cardiology unit through patient case studies which will focus on changes in practice made as a result of the agreed guidelines. This can be achieved by auditing standards of care (*Table 20.2*). Evaluation through auditing the infection rates of catheterised patients would be too complex a process because of the extrinsic factors that affect urinary tract infection rates (eg. in conditions such as diabetes).

Table 20.2: Standard in urinary catheters	
Standard statement	**Indicator**
All patients catheterised in Addenbrooke's NHS Trust are assessed and managed according to the guidelines	1. All nursing staff in Addenbrooke's NHS Trust have read the guidelines in catheter management
	2. All patients are assessed for need before the procedure and the Trust documentation form is placed in patient records
	3. All patients are catheterised using aseptic technique set out by Addenbrooke's NHS Trust policy
	4. The appropriate catheter and equipment is used: a. Catheter material b. Size of catheter and balloon size c. Drainage bag and stand/catheter valve
	5. All meatal cleansing is done daily with soap and water (Burke *et al*, 1981)
	6. All catheter bags are emptied individually using the correct procedure: a. Nurse washes hands before/after (Getliffe, 1996) b. Clean disposable gloves are worn c. Disposable containers (Crow *et al*, 1988)
	7. All catheters are removed at approximate time of midnight according to Addenbrooke's NHS Trust policy, unless otherwise indicated this demonstrates multiple, patient benefit (Crowe *et al*, 1993)

Primary outcomes

To date, the patient care primary outcomes are as follows:

1. The cardiology unit has stopped using several types of catheter and now only use the Bard Biocath™ hydrogel coated catheter because of its many advantages over other catheter types, especially for patients with haemodynamic instability (eg. myocardial infarction) (Talja *et al*, 1990) (cost of change is £24 per month).
2. A bedpan disposer has been installed, with the purpose of improving hygiene and preventing cross-infection (plastic urinals and bedpans are often not washed adequately).
3. Lignocaine gel is used accordingly to manufacturers' recommendations for both male and female patient catheterisation (Muctar, 1991).
4. All patient episodes of catheterisation are documented, including details of catheter used, clinician who carried out the procedure and length of time *in situ*.

With regard to the time taken to implement these changes to practice, the literature review took a week in total, including electronic and hand searching, telephoning, postal requests to other departments and companies and inter-library selection of papers. The critical analysis, criteria setting, prioritising and literature analysis took approximately 25 hours. The preparation and delivery of trust-wide presentations and two conference papers has been time-consuming. However, the cost has been offset by the benefits of the project, which include both the changes to practice and advertising the unit through dissemination of the work (*Table 20.3*).

The trust infection control team has collaborated in writing the hospital-wide guidelines. Ward staff are keen to see a change in practice. One of the positive responses has been that the project has conveyed a succinct message about 'best practice' and ideas about how much change is needed.

Difficulties associated with setting up the project

There have been difficulties associated with setting up the project as the cardiology medical staff did not consider the project high priority. In addition, management staff, although sympathetic, have not always given dedicated time for the work to be carried out and therefore it is progressing slowly. These examples of difficulties are entirely supported by the literature (ENB, 1996; Centre for Policy in Nursing Research, 1997).

Table 20.3: Financial cost of project *vs* benefits of project	
Financial cost of project (based on mid-scale F grade)	
One week F grade for literature review and critical analysis of papers	£375.00
One week F grade for writing up guidelines, working party meetings, etc.	£375.00
Two conference days F grade/conference fee and travel	£350.00
Four x 1/2 day F grade for Trust presentations	£150.00
Total	£1250.00
Benefits of project	
Changes in practice	
Raising profile of evidence-based practice	
Learning and appreciation of the process of evidence-based practice	
Advertising within Trust and nationally through presentations, conferences and publications	
Recruitment interest of staff through advertising	

The problems may be exacerbated by government and organisational pressures on staff to comply with evolving policy. The priority of the organisation is for clinicians to review and change practice but this is not always supported by an adequate infrastructure or resources. Sackett *et al* (1997) offer theoretical solutions to change in practice. However, the pressure to shift long-held prejudices of not only the medical profession but also many levels of management in the NHS should not always have to be borne by the clinical nursing staff.

The White Paper (DoH, 1998) gives a commitment to ensuring that the NHS is a universal service and discusses professional and patient 'partnerships' in care, but it does not provide the power base or framework within which nursing care can offer EBP. The RCN supports the opportunities that EBP can bring to nursing. However, the difficulties that the nursing staff experienced in achieving this small project provide an example of how hard it actually is to implement EBP.

On a more positive note, the care of patients in the cardiology unit in relation to urinary catheter management has been standardised and there is now evidence to support the change in practice; in addition, the quality of care is being monitored. Audit results are allied to standards of care and there is a predictability of outcomes from using specified interventions.

Conclusion

As a result of this work, staff in the NDU have devised a framework to monitor EBP projects which encourages the commitment of staff and a method of evaluating outcomes that are practice-based. The strategy is that staff will discuss an idea which is then committed to paper, eg. a summary of the project work, a planned outline and a business plan of the resources needed, and this is submitted to the planning team.

In response, the staff are given a contract with rostered and protected time, a project superviser is nominated who advises on frameworks, and experts are identified from whom staff can obtain information. This includes help with the research process, eg. identifying what effect the intended aims will have on practice, and help with evaluation.

Recommendations for staff have been summarised in *Table 20.4* with the aim that future work in EBP is given every opportunity for success through the creation of new supportive frameworks.

Table 20.4: Future recommendations
Appropriate project leader with working knowledge of evidence-based practice
Two to three people involved from outset, especially with responsibility for the literature review
Framework for project: checklist (Sackett *et al*, 1997); critique framework (Institute of Health Sciences, 1998)
Priority given for project: time, support, recognition
Involve all staff: to increase interest and motivation; ensure that change in practice is permanent
Be realistic in terms of time frames, eg. between one year and 18 months

Key points

❖ The cardiology nursing development unit (NDU) in Addenbrooke's NHS Trust Hospital designed a pilot project to experience the process of evidence-based practice (EBP).

❖ The aim was to provide a framework for EBP in order to guarantee success. This included: implementation and evaluation; the difficulties of EBP; and recommendations for staff.

❖ The NDU has now introduced a contract strategy for EBP.

❖ The subject for the pilot project was the management of urinary catheters, a patient-centred activity for which standards in care are now set and local guidelines produced.

❖ The infection control team and cardiology NDU are now devising hospital-wide guidelines in urinary catheter management.

References

Bard (1997) *Management and Care of Catheters and Collection Systems: A Guide for Nurses.*Bard, Crawley, West Sussex

Burke J, Garibaldi R, Britt M, Jacobson J, Conti M, Aling D (1981) Prevention of catheter associated urinary tract infection. *Am J Med* **70**: 655–8

Centre for Policy in Nursing Research (1997) *The NHS R&D Context for Nursing Research: A Working Paper.* London School of Hygiene and Tropical Medicine

Crow R, Mulhall A, Chapman R (1988) Indwelling catheterisation and related nursing practice. *J Adv Nurs* **13**: 489–95

Crowe H, Clift R, Douggon G, Bolton DM, Costello AJ (1993) Randomised study of the effect of midnight versus 0600 removal of urinary catheters. *Br J Urol* **71**: 306–8

DoH (1993) *Research for Health.* Department of Health, London

DoH (1998) *The New NHS: Modern, Dependable.* The Stationery Office, London

ENB (1996) *Teaching Research in Nursing and Midwifery Curricula* (Occasional report series). English National Board, London

ENB (1997) *Developing a Research Culture* (Occasional report series). English National Board, London

Getliffe K (1996) Care of urinary catheters. *Elder Care* April/May **8** (2): 23–29

Institute of Health Sciences (1998) *The Critical Appraisal Skills Programme.* Institute of Health Sciences, Old Road, Headington, Oxon OX8 7LF (Tel: 01865 226968)

Lewin K (1951) *Field Theory in Social Science.* Harper Row, New York

Marieb EN (1996) *Human Anatomy and Physiology.* 3rd edn. Benjamin Cummings, California

Muctar S (1991) The importance of a lubricant in transurethral interventions. *Urology* **31**: 153–5 (translation)

Sackett DL, Richardson WS, Rosenberg W, Haune RB (1997) *Evidence-based Medicine: How to Use Practice and Teach EBP.* Churchill Livingstone, Edinburgh

Talja M, Korpela A, Jarri K (1990) Comparison of urethral reaction to full silicone, hydrogen coated and silicone-latex catheters. *Br J Urol* **66**: 652–7

21

UTI in patients with urethral catheters: an audit tool

Patricia Penfold

This chapter presents an audit tool for the evaluation of practice relating to urinary tract infection in hospital patients with indwelling urethral catheters. It has been formulated primarily because urinary tract infection is a known complication of catheterisation, and because studies have shown practitioners' knowledge in this area to be poor. Although health professionals have an obligation to ensure their practice is evidence-based, this requires substantial time and skills in critical appraisal. The standard presented here is based on evidence from an extensive literature review on how best to minimise urinary tract infection during catheter insertion, meatal hygiene and management of the drainage system. The audit tool offers the potential for improved practice and demonstration of clinical effectiveness through measurable reduction in rates of urinary tract infection. Moreover, it provides an ideal opportunity for nurses to take the lead in clinical audit activity, which is so often medically led. The supplementary information will also provide a useful guide for nurses to undertake and initiate clinical audit activity in the future.

Urinary tract infections (UTIs) are a major complication of urethral catheterisation (Hart, 1985; Gooch, 1986; Wright, 1988; Roe, 1993; Stickler and Zimakoff, 1994; Winn, 1996). Aseptic catheter insertion and effective catheter care — meatal hygiene, washing hands before emptying catheter bags, and maintenance of a closed urine drainage system — are important factors in minimising the occurrence of UTI. Poor catheter insertion and catheter care techniques have a significant impact on the development of UTI, which can have serious consequences such as renal damage and death (Hart, 1985; Roe, 1993).

Despite this, studies indicate a poor level of knowledge among nurses on catheter selection (Crummey, 1989; Henry, 1992), catheter care and education of patients (Roe, 1989; Carson and Culyer, 1996). A study carried out to assess competency of doctors in catheterisation found considerable ignorance of the practical and theoretical aspects, suggesting that doctors were inadequately taught this procedure (Carter *et al*, 1990). Clearly prevention of catheter-acquired infection is a significant challenge to the multidisciplinary team.

Clinical audit

Quality patient care is indicated by the delivery of evidence-based practice (EBP). Health professionals have an obligation to ensure they are providing the best patient care available, and that care is proven to be effective (Humphris and Littlejohns, 1995). It is not enough to merely implement EBP, the effects of interventions need to be evaluated to ensure best practice is actually being delivered. For clinical effectiveness to be demonstrated, the impact of changed practice needs to be evaluated, and improved patient outcome shown as a result (McClarey and Duff, 1997).

Although clinicians are used to assessing and evaluating health care, this is rarely 'systematic, critical analysis of the quality of care, including the procedures used for diagnosis and treatment, the use of resources and the resulting outcome and quality of life for the patient', which define audit (Department of Health, 1989). Clinical audit is one example of an activity within the umbrella of clinical governance, which aims to ensure clinicians are improving and maintaining the quality of their care. NHS trusts have an obligation to prove that they are using processes, such as clinical audit, which guarantee quality assurance (Garbett, 1998).

Clinical audit is an excellent tool to implement best practice because it demands a clear definition of the level of quality to be attained and uses a process that enables practitioners to examine, reflect on and improve their own practice (Kinn, 1995). It also enables the evaluation of the effects of interventions, which is an essential part of clinical effectiveness (Ross, 1996). It is for this reason that a clinical audit tool has been chosen for this subject.

Many nurses lack confidence in carrying out and using research and audit (Kinn, 1995; Hicks, 1997), believing that the nursing contribution to care does not make a real difference to patient outcomes, despite growing evidence to the contrary (Kitson, 1997). The tool presented in this chapter is simple enough to be incorporated into routine clinical practice, and the potential for the relatively quick demonstration of improved outcomes should help maintain interest and build confidence (Kinn, 1995). The tool also provides an ideal opportunity for nurses to take the lead in clinical audit activity, which is so often medically led (Malby, 1995).

The aim of clinical audit is to review clinical practice and implement change in order to meet a set target (Birkett, 1995). The target is the level of quality to be attained, and is defined in the form of standards, criteria or guidelines. These are formed from evidence (such as research) of what constitutes best practice (Harvey, 1996).

Evidence-based practice

EBP uses a hierarchy of evidence sometimes described as levels. The idea is to start looking for evidence at the top (first) level, and to keep going down the hierarchy until the best evidence available is found.

First-level evidence involves the identification of all research in a specific area, appraisal and analysis of its quality, and summarising the relevant findings into recommendations or guidelines for clinical practice. Organisations that produce such evidence are the UK Cochrane Centre and the NHS Centre for Reviews and Dissemination. Neither were able to find clinical guidelines for catheter management.

Second-level evidence includes systematic reviews and overviews of appraised research. The Cochrane database, available in all NHS organisations, keeps a record of second-level evidence that is judged to be of sound quality. A search of this produced no second-level evidence, but many useful references for third-level evidence, which is sound original research. Third-level evidence was also found by contacting the Nursing and Midwifery Audit and Information Centre and the National Centre for Clinical Audit, and by searching the Medline and CINAHL databases.

Once all the suggested references had been retrieved they needed to be critically appraised. There were some literature reviews on catheter management, but as these had not already been appraised (by the Cochrane Centre, for example), it was difficult to ascertain how systematic they actually were. Indications of the extent of critical appraisal, such as the quality of the academic journal, the volume and scope of research reviewed, and evidence within the text of critical appraisal, were used to determine how rigorous they were.

Many of the references turned out to be unsound research or fourth-level evidence. Fourth-level evidence is anecdotal evidence or expert opinion. It can also be the results of quality improvement programmes, such as the clinical guidelines on preventing catheter-related infections in hospital patients formulated by the Public Health Laboratory Service (PHLS) (Ward *et al*, 1997). Although these guidelines are based on the results of a large multidisciplinary audit over 19 hospitals, the authors acknowledge that they did not undertake the full process of guideline production, which includes a literature review followed by dissemination, implementation, evaluation and review of the guidelines in practice. EBP places less importance on fourth-level evidence than experimental research, but there may be limitations with this (Kitson, 1997).

Nursing has not yet accrued an extensive body of experimental research and many nursing interventions are not capable of being examined with the type of rigour demanded by scientific research (Kitson, 1997; White, 1997). It is only recently that the contribution of the multidisciplinary team in influencing patient outcomes has been recognised. The reliance on pharmacological or medical interventions in measuring outcomes ignores the contribution that the rest of the multidisciplinary team may have made (Kitson, 1997). Fourth-level evidence may therefore be important, and the PHLS guidelines have been included as evidence.

Preparation for clinical audit

Multidisciplinary audit is essential in order to look at the overall picture of quality of care, and because people or groups in organisations do not work in isolation. The essence of clinical audit is that it is concerned with improvements in care for the patient (Baker *et al*, 1995).

A truly patient-focused approach is only possible by considering the different perspectives of all those involved in care delivery. Clinical audit must therefore be a multidisciplinary venture, with clear roles and responsibilities allocated to members of the multidisciplinary team (Greenhalgh and Fairfield, 1996).

The multidisciplinary team need to decide whether they are prepared to commit themselves to undertaking clinical audit, as the audit process may highlight problems in team collaboration. Some teambuilding may be necessary before the audit can begin. The use of a facilitator is acknowledged as a useful resource in guiding and supporting the team and ensuring that no one group 'owns' the audit (Ross, 1996). A member of the clinical audit or nursing development department might be prepared to take on this role. McClarey and Duff (1997) recommend incorporating audit activity into existing social settings and forums to enable team members to discuss and debate proposed change. This is important in ensuring that the team feels involved and not threatened (Kinn, 1995).

Leadership is one of the key factors in the success of audit (Harvey, 1996). Opinion leaders are individuals who are clinically credible and have the ability to lead others (McClarey and Duff, 1997). An infection control nurse, clinical nurse specialist or continence adviser may be suitable for this role.

Different leaders may also emerge at the different stages of the audit process. A facilitator can again be useful in identifying members' strengths in relation to particular tasks (Morrell and Harvey, 1996).

Clinical audit cannot be viewed in isolation, but needs to be part of the organisation's overall quality strategy (Øvretveit, 1992; Ross, 1996). The occurrence of UTI has economic implications such as increased time spent in hospital (Hart, 1985). Effective use of resources is an important part of clinical effectiveness, and is highly relevant to the organisation as a whole. It is therefore important that managers are involved in the clinical audit process, as they may have more authority to effect necessary changes (Exworthy, 1996): many hospital hierarchies still place nurses in a reactive rather than a proactive role (Hunt, 1987). However, it is important that clinical audit remains clinician led, as most aspects of clinical quality can only be effectively assessed and improved by clinicians themselves (Øvretveit, 1992).

The clinical audit model

The audit model described by Redfern and Norman (1996) has been chosen because it is clearly set out, easy to understand and reflects the key principles of clinical audit. It uses the following framework.

Identifying the issue to be audited

This has already been discussed.

Setting the standard

A standard consists of a specific statement of quality that can be measured. The standard should define the quality of care a patient can expect to receive and the outcome for the patient (Malby, 1995; West and Lyon, 1995). The standard in *Figure 21.1* has been formulated following an extensive review of the evidence concerning UTI in catheterised patients. A generalised statement about the overall quality feature of catheter management has been used (Øvretveit, 1992), followed by specific measurable standards, the first of which concerns UTI. This allows the quality statement to be built on as more evidence is gathered about other aspects of catheter management (such as prevention of catheter blockage), and other standards created at a later date.

Between 16% and 35% of hospital patients with indwelling catheters develop UTIs (Hart, 1985; Roe, 1985; Wright, 1988; Hustinx *et al*, 1991), with infection being defined as 10^5 or more colony forming units (cfu) of bacteria per ml of urine (Kass, 1956). Risk of infection increases the longer the catheter is *in situ* (Hart, 1985), with most hospital patients being catheterised for less than seven days (Stickler and Zimakoff, 1994).

A standard needs to be realistic; if it is too high it may lead to disillusionment (Kinn, 1995). For example, a 0% incidence of infection is unrealistic, because even with the most stringent practice, some patients will develop infection (Hustinx *et al*, 1991). The standard therefore reflects the most widely used prevalence figure of 23% (Kunin and McCormack, 1966) (see *Figure 21.1*). A similar standard is advocated by Wyatt and Timoney (1987).

Whatever the outcome measure, there needs to be a measure of the interventions that influence it in order to examine and improve them (Mead, 1996). Generally the standard statement is supplemented by criteria, which identify what is necessary for the successful achievement of the standard. A well known approach is to organise the criteria into resources or equipment (structure), actions or decisions (process) and results (outcomes) (Kitson, 1989).

According to Hart (1985), there are three ways in which bacteria can enter the bladder in catheterised patients:

- on insertion of the catheter
- via the junction of the catheter with the meatal area
- via the drainage system.

Patients with indwelling urethral catheters will receive best clinical practice in catheter management as demonstrated by:		
Standard 1: The overall incidence of urinary tract infections in patients with indwelling urethral catheters will not exceed 23%		
Structure	**Process**	**Outcome**
1.Catheter insertion Clinicians will receive education on catheter insertion. Sterile catheterisation packs and equipment, antiseptic wash will be available.	Antiseptic handwash will be used before and following catheterisation. Meatal area will be cleansed with sterile saline or water before catheterisation. Aseptic technique will be used.	Clinicians will understand and apply the principles of effective catheter insertion and aseptic techniques.
2. Meatal hygiene Clinicians will receive education in the principles of meatal hygiene.	Meatal/catheter junction will be cleansed with soap and water during patient's normal hygiene routine.	Meatal/catheter junction will be free of encrustations.
3. Management of drainage system Clinicians will receive education in the principles of managing a closed drainage system. Sterile catheter bags, disposal gloves and chlorhexidine wipes will be available. Bedpan washer or sterile jugs will be available.	Drainage system will be kept closed except to empty drainage bag twice daily, or to change bag if damaged, leaking, smelling or sediment is present. Emptying bags — hands will be washed and drainage port swabbed with chlorhexidine before and after emptying. Disposable gloves will be worn. Receptacle used will be sterile, or have been washed in bedpan washer and dried.	Clinicians will understand and apply the principles of management of the closed drainage system.

Figure 21.1: Quality standard statement on indwelling urethral catheters

The criteria in the standard (*Figure 21.1*) describe the interventions needed to minimise infection via these three routes, based on the following evidence.

Catheter insertion: Insertion of the catheter should be aseptic (Hart, 1985; Roe, 1985; Wyatt and Timoney, 1987), with an antiseptic handwash used before the procedure (Wyatt and Timoney, 1987; Ehrenkranz and Alfonso, 1991). Some evidence suggests that disinfection of the urethra before catheterisation with a solution such as chlorhexidine reduces the risk of UTI (Roe, 1985; Wright, 1988; Gould, 1994). More recently, the use of chlorhexidine has been questioned because of the possible emergence of resistant organisms (Roe, 1993) and the risk of trauma to delicate urethral tissue (Gould, 1994). The PHLS recommendations to cleanse the urethral area with sterile saline or water are therefore recommended (Ward *et al*, 1997). Even more important than urethral cleansing is practitioner competence in the technique of catheter insertion (Hart, 1985; Roe, 1985).

There is little evidence relating catheter material or size to infection. Catheters with a hydrogel-type coating may be more resistant to bacterial colonisation (Wilde, 1997), although there is no conclusive evidence to support this. The issues of catheter selection and frequency of changing should form the basis of a subsequent standard, as there is much more evidence relating them to problems such as catheter blockage, leakage, bladder spasm, urethral inflammation and stricture formation (Roe, 1985; Getliffe, 1994a; Wilde, 1997).

Meatal hygiene: This is a controversial area. Some evidence suggests that it may not play an important part in the development of infection (Hart, 1985). Most studies have been uncontrolled or used small samples (Roe, 1985). Of two large controlled studies carried out, one found meatal hygiene with antiseptic solutions to be ineffective (Classen *et al*, 1991), while the other found that it may actually increase the risk of infection (Burke *et al*, 1981). Ward *et al* (1997) suggest performing meatal care at intervals appropriate for keeping the meatus free of encrustations. Anecdotal evidence suggests washing the meatal area with soap and water as part of normal hygiene routines.

Management of the drainage system: Maintenance of a closed system of drainage is essential for management of indwelling catheters (Hart, 1985; Roe, 1985; Wyatt and Timoney, 1987). Disconnection or opening of the closed drainage system should be kept to a minimum (Hart, 1985; Wyatt and Timoney, 1987), although how often it should be opened to allow emptying of the drainage bag is unclear. There is some evidence to recommend twice a day (Roe, 1985), but care will need to be taken to ensure bags do not become overfull. Although no reliable studies have been carried out, anecdotal evidence suggests that gloves are worn to empty drainage bags, and that a dry receptacle is used that is either sterile or has been washed with detergent and hot water (Roe, 1985; Ward *et al*, 1997). The port of the drainage bag should be swabbed with chlorhexidine before and after emptying (Roe, 1985; Ward *et al*, 1997).

The use of chlorhexidine in the bag itself is of no proven benefit (Roe, 1985; Wright, 1988; Gillespie *et al*, 1983). In the absence of evidence as to frequency of bag changes, Ward *et al* (1997) advocate changing the bag if it is damaged, leaking, smelling or there is an accumulation of sediment.

There is some evidence that bladder installations may be effective in preventing catheter blockage in long-term catheterisation (Getliffe, 1994b). However, care practices relating to prevention of infection are unrelated to incidence of catheter blockage (Getliffe, 1994a). The use of bladder installations or washouts is therefore inappropriate in relation to prevention of UTI, but may be of benefit in a standard related to prevention of catheter blockage.

To prevent cross-infection, hands should be washed and dried before and after handling the catheter or drainage bags (Hart, 1985; Roe, 1985). Although some evidence suggests that catheterised patients should be nursed in separate rooms (Roe, 1985), other evidence conflicts with this (Hart, 1985), and in practice this would be difficult to carry out.

In the absence of large-scale trials, the effect of prophylactic antibiotics in preventing infection is inconclusive (Hustinx *et al*, 1991; Roe, 1993). The best way of avoiding catheter-associated UTI is to avoid insertion of catheters wherever possible (Hart, 1985; Roe, 1985; Stickler and Zimakoff, 1994; Ward *et al*, 1997). Guidelines on the indications for catheterisation should be incorporated into the overall catheter management strategy.

Measuring the quality and checking the results against the standard set

This part of the audit cycle involves the assessment of current practice compared with the standard and criteria outcomes specified in *Figure 21.1*. The processes should not be implemented until this baseline information has been collected, to allow accurate comparison of practice before and after their implementation (Kinn, 1995).

It is important to choose a method of data collection that is appropriate to the audit. Occurrence screening, which uses a specific clinical indicator as a measure of outcome, is a good method of measuring infection rates (Bennett and Walshe, 1990; Hartigan, 1995). Each patient who is catheterised has a proforma, which documents urinalysis or urine microscopy on insertion and removal of the catheter, at weekly intervals and at any other time if clinical symptoms of infection develop as suggested by Crummey (1985) and Wyatt and Timoney (1987) (*Figure 21.2*). Clinical symptoms of infection are pyrexia, dysuria or general malaise. Urine specimens should be collected and analysed and the proformas filled in. The correct method of specimen collection is crucial to avoid contamination of the urine (Sussman, 1990). Correct technique is to use a sterile needle and syringe inserted into the sampling sleeve of the catheter bag, and to withdraw a small amount of urine and deposit it in a sterile universal container.

Patient name ....
Hospital number ....
Ward ....
CATHETER INSERTION
Date.................................. Urinalysis.................................... Microscopy result (if applicable)
....
CATHETER REMOVAL
Date .... Urinalysis.................................... Microscopy result (if applicable)
....
WEEKLY URINALYSIS
Date .... Urinalysis.................................... Microscopy result (if applicable)
....
....
SYMPTOMS OF URINARY TRACT INFECTION
Date .... Urinalysis.................................... Microscopy result (if applicable)
....

Figure 21.2: Urinary tract infection screening: patient proforma

Any urine infections (10^5cfu or more per ml of urine) should be treated with antibiotics. Each separate episode of infection should be treated as an occurrence. A representative patient sample needs to be obtained rather than a statistically significant one, as the object is to collect enough data to inform and evaluate the change process (Harvey, 1996). Data collection should continue for as long as the multidisciplinary team think it is necessary.

Urinalysis reagent strips, which screen for nitrites, leucocytes, blood and protein, avoid the costly practice of sending all urine specimens for microscopy, as only specimens that are positive to any of the four need be sent. Urine that is negative to all four can safely be assumed to be free from infection (Sussman, 1990; Laker, 1994).

The disadvantage of occurence screening is that it is difficult to attribute outcomes to clinical practice (West and Lyon, 1995). It should therefore not be the only method used. Criterion-based audit measures quality using the structure, processes and outcomes on which the standard is based (Hartigan, 1995). This will often mean focusing on staff performance (West and Lyon, 1995). Questionnaires or direct observation would both be suitable for assessing staff performance, but direct observation is very threatening. Anonymous questionnaires, which assess clinicians' knowledge of catheter management, are therefore suggested.

A common problem with these is not asking the appropriate questions. The suggested example questionnaire in *Figure 21.3* is based closely on the standard criteria, and uses unambiguous 'yes/no' questions where possible (West and Lyon, 1995). However, some open questions are included to find out the reasons for problems and where specific answers are needed.

The audit tool should be valid (accurately measure what it sets out to) and reliable (consistent) (Kinn *et al*, 1995). It is recommended that a pilot of the audit tool is carried out before the audit begins. This should help highlight any ambiguities with the tool, and allow adaptation of the questionnaire or patient proforma as appropriate in order to ensure validity and reliability each time they are used.

Identifying whether any change is needed

Following data collection and analysis, the results should be constructively fed back to the multidisciplinary group, highlighting areas of good practice and areas needing improvement. A great deal of sensitivity and trust is needed at this point (Morrell and Harvey, 1996). It is likely that clinicians will not be fully aware or using the correct principles of aseptic technique and catheter management. Their comments from the questionnaires should help to determine why.

Deciding strategies for change

The whole multidisciplinary group needs to be involved in deciding strategies for change. These include agreeing on the appropriate courses of action, who is responsible for action, and the timescale for implementing the changes and reauditing (Morrell and Harvey, 1996). This may mean setting up educational sessions.

Guidelines for practice, based on the evidence presented in this chapter, could be created. Organisational change involving other departments, eg. pharmacy, supplies or microbiology, may be needed.

Please circle your answer, and comment where appropriate		
1a	Do you wash your hands with antiseptic handwash before inserting a catheter?	Yes/No
1b	If no what are your reasons?	
2a	Do you use a sterile catheterisation pack?	Yes/No
2b	If no what are your reasons?	
3a	Do you use sterile equipment, eg. gloves and catheter?	Yes/No
3b	If no what are your reasons?	
4a	Do you clean the meatal area with sterile saline or water before inserting the catheter?	Yes/No
4b	If no what are your reasons?	
5a	Have you received education in the principles in aseptic techniques?	Yes/No
5b	Do you understand the principles of aseptic technique?	Yes/No
6	Have you received education on male catheterisation?	Yes/No
7	Have you received education on female catheterisation?	Yes/No
8a	What do you use to clean the meatal/catheter junction?	Yes/No
8b	How often do you clean the meatal/catheter junction?	Yes/No
9a	Do you wash your hands before emptying a catheter bag?	Yes/No
9b	Do you wash your hands after emptying a catheter bag?	Yes/No
10a	Do you wear disposable gloves to empty a catheter bag?	Yes/No
10b	If no what are your reasons?	
11a	Do you swab the port of the catheter bag with chlorhexidine before and after emptying it?	Yes/No
11b	If no what are your reasons?	
12a	To empty the catheter bag, do you use a receptacle that is either sterile or has been washed in a bedpan washer and dried immediately before use?	Yes/No
12b	If no what are your reasons?	
13	How often do you empty the catheter bag?	Yes/No
14a	Do you ever change the catheter bag?	Yes/No
14b	If yes, what are your reasons?	
15a	Apart from changing the catheter bag, do you ever disconnect the catheter from the drainage bag?	Yes/No
15b	If yes, what are your reasons?	
16	Do you understand the principles of management of the closed drainage system?	Yes/No

Figure 21.3: Questionnaire: management of urethral catheters

Implementing necessary changes

No matter how well the multidisciplinary team works together, there may be resistance to implementing new ideas. Collaboration, consultation and multiprofessional agreement are necessary at every stage (McClarey and Duff, 1997). Someone within the team with an interest in or knowledge of urinary problems, such as a continence link nurse, may be a useful and credible link to facilitate the change process. A facilitator is also a good resource at this stage (Kinn, 1995). Early groundwork to ensure that the multidisciplinary team is prepared for audit is important for successful implementation later on.

Monitoring the effect of the change against the standard

Reaudit is essential to see if the changes implemented have met the standard.

Encouragement and support need to be given to the multidisciplinary team; even if the standard has not been met, it will hopefully be possible to see improvements when comparing results with the first audit. Audit should be an ongoing activity, and reaudit is necessary to ensure that the standard is met or continues to be maintained (Kinn, 1995; Morrell and Harvey, 1996).

Conclusion

This chapter has presented a clinical audit tool for evaluation of practice relating to urinary infection rates in hospital patients with indwelling urethral catheters. In an area where there may be confusion and ignorance, it states the evidence on which to base clinical practice in techniques of catheter insertion, meatal hygiene and management of the closed drainage system, and offers the potential to demonstrate improved patient outcomes. It is also hoped that clear demonstration of how the tool was created will help provide clinical nurses with the knowledge and skills to undertake and lead clinical audit activity in the future.

Key points

- ❖ Urinary tract infection (UTI) is a serious complication of urethral catheterisation.

- ❖ Studies have shown that practitioners' knowledge and techniques in the selection, care and insertion of catheters and the education of patients is poor.

- ❖ Practitioners have an obligation to base practical interventions on reliable evidence, but this demands time and appraisal skills.

- ❖ The standard and audit tool presented here demonstrates evidence-based care practices which should ensure catheter-related UTI is kept to a minimum, and that quality care is maintained.

References

Baker R, Sorrie R, Reddish S, Hearnshaw H, Robertson N (1995) The facilitation of multiprofessional clinical audit in primary health care teams — from audit to quality assurance. *J Int Care* **9**(3): 237–44
Bennett J, Walshe K (1990) Occurrence screening as a method of audit. *Br Med J* **300**: 1248–51
Birkett M (1995) Is audit action research? *Physiotherapy* **81**(4): 190–4
Burke J, Garibaldi R, Britt M, Jacobson J, Conti M, Alling D (1981) Prevention of catheter-associated urinary tract infections. Efficacy of daily meatal care regimens. *Am J Med* **70**(3): 655–8
Carson M, Culyer L (1996) Catheter care. *Primary Health Care* **6**(6): 17–19
Carter R, Aithison M, Mufti G, Scott R (1990) Catheterisation: your urethra in their hands. *Br Med J* **301**: 905

Classen D, Larsen R, Burke J, Alling D, Stevens L (1991) Daily meatal care for prevention of catheter-associated bacteriuria: results using frequent applications of polyantibiotic cream. *Infect Control Hosp Epidemiol* **12**(3): 151–62

Crummey V (1985) Hospital-acquired urinary tract infection. *Nurs Times* **81**(5 June) (suppl): 7–12

Crummey V (1989) Ignorance can hurt. *Nurs Times* **85**(21): 66–7

Department of Health (1989) *Working for Patients. Medical Audit.* Working Paper 6. HMSO, London

Ehrenkranz N, Alfonso B (1991) Failure of bland soap handwash to prevent hand transfer of patient bacteria to urethral catheters. *Infect Control Hosp Epidemiol* **12**(11): 654–62

Exworthy M (1996) Managers and clinical audit: past, present and future. *Br J Healthcare Management* **2**: 605–8

Garbett R (1998) Clinical governance? *Nurs Times* **2**(7): 15

Getliffe K (1994a) The characteristics and management of patients with long-term urinary catheters. *J Adv Nurs* **20**(1): 140–9

Getliffe K (1994b) The use of bladder washouts to reduce urinary catheter encrustation. *Br J Urol* **73**(6): 696–700

Gillespie W, Jones J, Teasdale C, Simpson R, Nashep L, Speller D (1983) Does the addition of disinfectant to urine drainage bags prevent infection in catheterised patients? *Lancet* **i**: 1037–9

Gooch J (1986) Catheter care. *Profess Nurse* **1**(8): 207–8

Gould D (1994) Keeping on tract. *Nurs Times* **90**(40): 58–64

Greenhalgh J, Fairfield G (1996) Outcomes and audit into practice. *Outcomes Briefing* **7**: 32–5

Hart J (1985) The urethral catheter — a review of its implication in urinary tract infection. *Nurs Studies* **22**(1): 57–70

Hartigan G (1995) Choosing a method for clinical audit: the first hurdle. *Physiotherapy* **81**(4): 187–8

Harvey G (1996) Relating quality assessment and audit to the research process in nursing. *Nurse Researcher* **3**(3): 35–45

Henry M (1992) Catheter confusion. *Nurs Times* **88**(42): 65–72

Hicks C (1997) The dilemma of incorporating research into clinical practice. *Br J Nurs* **6**(9): 511–15

Humphris D, Littlejohns P (1995) The development of multiprofessional audit and clinical guidelines: their contribution to quality assurance and effectiveness in the NHS. *J Interprofessional Care* **9**(3): 207–25

Hunt M (1987) The process of translating research findings into nursing practice. *J Adv Nurs* **12**: 101–10

Hustinx W, Mintjes-De Groot R, Verkooyen R, Verbrugh H (1991) Impact of concurrent antimicrobial therapy on catheter-associated urinary tract infection. *J Hosp Infection* **18**(1): 45–56

Kass EH (1956) Asymptomatic infections of the urinary tract. *Transactions of the Association of American Physicians* **69**: 56–63

Kinn S (1995) Clinical audit — a tool for nursing practice. *Nurs Standard* **9**(4): 35–6

Kinn S, Semple E, Hillan E (1995) *The Audit Handbook for Professions Allied to Medicine.* Glasgow University, Glasgow

Kitson A (1989) *A Framework for Quality. A Patient-Centred Approach to Quality Assurance in Health Care.* RCN Standards of Care Project. Scutari, London

Kitson A (1997) Using evidence to demonstrate the value of nursing. *Nurs Standard* **11**(28): 34–9

Kunin C, McCormack R (1966) Prevention of catheter-induced urinary tract infection by sterile closed drainage. *New Engl J Med* **274**: 1155–61

Laker C (1994) Urological investigations. In: Laker C, ed. *Urological Nursing.* Scutari, London: 37–65

McClarey M, Duff L (1997) Clinical effectiveness and evidence-based practice. *Nurs Standard* **11**(52): 33–7

Malby R (1995) *Clinical Audit for Nurses and Therapists.* Scutari, London

Mead D (1996) Research-based tools in the audit process: issues of use, validity and reliability. *Nurse Researcher* **3**(3): 17–34

Morrell C, Harvey G (1996) Clinical audit. *Nurs Standard* **10**(17): 38–42

Øvretveit J (1992) *Health Service Quality. An Introduction to Quality Methods for Health Services.* Blackwell Scientific Publications, Oxford

Redfern S, Norman J (1996) Clinical audit, related cycles and types of health care quality: a preliminary model. *Int J Qual Health Care* **8**(4): 331–40

Roe B (1985) Catheter care: an overview. *Int J Nurs Studies* **22**: 45–56

Roe B (1989) Study of information given by nurses for catheter care to patients and their carers. *J Adv Nurs* **14**(3): 203–10

Roe B (1993) Catheter-associated urinary tract infection: a review. *J Clin Nurs* **2**(4): 197–203

Ross F (1996) Interprofessional audit: the need for teamwork when researching quality of care. *Nurse Researcher* **3**(3): 47–57

Stickler D, Zimakoff J (1994) Complications of urinary tract infections associated with devices used for long-term bladder management. *J Hosp Infection* **28**: 177–94

Sussman M (1990) Urinary tract infection: an overview. In: Newall R, Howell R, eds. *Clinical Urinalysis. The Principle and Practice of Urine Testing in the Hospital and Community*. Stoke Poges, Buckinghamshire: 50–61

Ward V, Wilson J, Taylor L, Cookson B, Glynn A (1997) *Preventing Hospital-Acquired Infection.* Public Health Laboratory Service, London

West B, Lyon M (1995) Surgical nurse principles of audit and clinical practice. *Br J Nurs* **4**(17): 987–91

White S (1997) Evidence-based practice and nursing: the new panacea? *Br J Nurs* **6**(3): 175–8

Wilde M (1997) Long-term indwelling urinary catheter care: conceptualising the research base. *J Adv Nurs* **25**: 1252–61

Winn C (1996) Basing catheter care on research principles. *Nurs Standard* **10**(18): 38–40

Wright E (1988) Catheter care: the risk of infection. *Profess Nurse* **3**(12): 487–8, 490

Wyatt T, Timoney R (1987) The effect of introducing a policy of catheter care on the infection rate in a small hospital. *J Hosp Infection* **9**: 230–4